Many pe[illegible]
graduate students can take [illegible]age from [illegible]
reflected in these chapters and from the ways that phenomenology can be used as a method for nursing inquiry. More importantly, the subject matter brings into sharp relief issues that practitioners encounter regularly but which they may no longer really notice. This is a book about the experience of the patient as 'other' and the care which they recieve in pain and distress and when they suffer from unpleasant conditions. This is the domain in which nurses claim a special place. This work puts that claim under the spotlight.

Jocalyn Lawler RN PhD
Professor of Nursing, University of Sydney

Nurses have always known that by understanding the experience of illness and being cared for, we become better nurses, better able to provide appropriate care. This volume makes an extraordinary contribution in this area, providing insight into the experience and meaning of being a patient.

The first two chapters provide context for the phenomenological approach to the research, and in the type of understanding that phenomenological inquiry provides for nursing. The remaining seven chapters provide wonderful insights into being a patient: the experience of illness, of receiving care in various situations. They are exquisitely crafted stories prepared by an extraordinary group of international authors. Their research depicts the experiences and meaning of living with schizophrenia, leg ulcers, breast cancer and mastectomy, of chronic pain and inflicted pain.

This book is essential reading for the beginning nurse (as an introduction to the patient's world), as well as the experienced nurse (as their patients are people). Reading this book will help us all become richer, wiser, a better person and a better nurse.

Janice M. Morse, PhD (Nurs), PhD (Anthro), FAAN
Director, International Institute for Qualitative Methodology,
University of Alberta

NURSING AND THE EXPERIENCE OF ILLNESS

Phenomenology in Practice

Edited by

IRENA MADJAR & JO ANN WALTON

with a foreword by Max van Manen

ROUTLEDGE
London and New York

First published in 1999 by Routledge
11 New Fetter Lane, London EC4P 4EE

Simultaneously published in the USA and Canada
by Routledge
29 West 35th Street, New York, NY 10001

Set in 10/12pt Goudy Old Style by DOCUPRO, Sydney
Printed by KHL Printing Co. Pte Ltd, Singapore

British Library Cataloguing in Publication Data
A catalogue record for this book is available from the British Library

Library of Congress Cataloging in Publication Data
A catalogue record for this book has been requested

ISBN 0-415-20782-7 (hbk)
ISBN 0-415-20783-5 (pbk)

Foreword

MAX VAN MANEN

In the first chapter of this book Jo Ann Walton and Irena Madjar refer to the phenomenological stance as 'the listening gaze'. The phrase 'the listening gaze' provides an appropriate starting point from which to comment on the ambition of this Australian work. As a methodological expression 'the listening gaze' is not only indicative of doing phenomenological research, it is also expressive of the visitor's experience of Australia—a land of wondrous exoticism and of people who stand in a sensual-sensible relation to their habitat.

The listening gaze. There seems to be a passive, receptive quality to the coupling 'listening' and 'gaze'. In a way this passivity captures nicely the questioning, wondering mood of phenomenological thought. Nowadays the spirit of activism too frequently seems to have overtaken the spirit of patient thinking, quiet wondering. In fact, the greatest hindrance to gaining access to the phenomenology of wonder and thoughtful reflection is perhaps our cultural inclination to devalue passivity in favour of a pervasive activism in all realms of inquiry. Could it be that we are so inclined to convert research into action (as the appeal of the term 'action research' attests) that this activism can limit our possibility for understanding?

But, to be sure, the phrase 'the listening gaze' has also more dynamic signification. Whenever or wherever we look our gaze is always interested, attentive, selective, preoccupied with something. Similarly, when we hear something then our listening is attentive, selective. Phenomenology has shown that vision and hearing are experientially complex: when we gaze at something then our ears, our skin, our motility and our linguisticality are also involved in this seeing. Understanding arises precisely in the mutual partaking of our various sensibilities. Thus, when we walk along a beautiful sunny Australian beach we 'see' the sand and the ocean with the sensuality of our skin, we 'feel' the wide expanse with the attunement of our ears, and we 'hear' the crashing of the rolling waves with our eyes. Ordinary experience confirms what Van den Berg (1972) suggested some 50 years ago—that we feel with our eyes, touch with our words, and that sometimes it may even happen that our ears make us see, such as when we hear a lengthy parade go by, too loud with noisy marching bands. We do not have to look at the marching bands because, in our desire for some quiet calm, our ears already 'see' too much.

It may also happen that a sound is so strangely overwhelming that it disturbs our seeing, and thereby makes our environment strange, hostile or disorienting. During a visit to the Australian North-East, I was driven in the car of my host to the university campus which is located in what Australians call 'the bush'. I was completely unprepared for what happened to me when I opened the door and stepped out of the car. Met by an incredible screaming that burst forth from the trees around us, I was startled, not knowing what was going on. Crickets? No, these could not be just crickets. This piercing chirping sound was just too immense, too totally penetrating. It had the metalic ring of a million electrical high-power wires. And yet, I could not see what my ears were telling me. Something in those gangly trees, those burnt bushes, that red-hot sand which surrounded me there hovered a wild noise that I could not shut out, from which I could not turn away.

My first impulse was to get back into the car to get away from this alarming sound, but then my host reassured me. The deafening shrill squeal was neither threatening nor artificial. These were the love songs of the cicadas. Thousands and thousands of cicadas. They had emerged from their seven-year burial, clinging to the bark of trees where they were to undergo a metamorphic transformation, leaving their hard body shells tacked to tree trunks, like frozen soldiers—and now their fate was to sing without eating until death.

My host smiled—she was used to the summer sounds of the Australian bush. But I had trouble shaking off the totally bewitching effect of that deafening, piercing, shrill call of the cicadas. It was as if my eyes needed to believe my ears, to make comprehensible what they could not fathom by themselves. This listening interfered with my gaze.

Later it occurred to me that these were the same cicadas that

Socrates must have been talking about in his dialogue with Phaedrus, when their topic of conversation turned to the persuasive and enchanting quality of certain kinds of writing. Socrates and Phaedrus go for a stroll in the country where the cicadas, like the mythological Sirens, are singing their bewitching songs in the trees above their heads. The philosopher explains to Phaedrus that according to legend cicadas were once human; young men who had fallen under the spell of the Muses when they first visited the earth. The men were so ravished by the sweetness of the songs of the Muses that in their devotion to the singing maidens they took no thought of food or drink. And so they died before they knew what was happening to them. From them sprang thereafter the cicadas to whom the Muses granted the privilege that they should be allowed to sing from the moment of birth until death, without the need to eat or drink.

The reason that Socrates recounts the myth of the cicadas is to point out that language too can have this bewitching effect—for good or for bad. Words too affect how and what we see and feel. The sophists, contemporaries of Socrates, were known for their persuasive speeches, rhetoric, with which they could cast a spell on their audience. In this dialogue, Socrates and Phaedrus are actually discussing the meaning of love: true love as opposed to the physical love that Phaedrus had found in the writings of Lysias. Socrates points out that the mere rhetoric of written speeches cannot do justice to the living meaning of life's passions; and so their conversation turns into the famous question of the virtue of the written word.

How do the issues of the bewitching songs of the cicadas, the sensibility of understanding, the value of writing, and the relation between language and experience speak to this Australian text of the phenomenology of nursing? The encounter with the cicadas may remind us of the fact that we live in different worlds. For many people experiences such as chronic pain, schizophrenia or mastectomy, do not belong to their lifeworld. Other people suffer from these conditions but they may not really understand them. Still others (practitioners of the health sciences) have 'knowledge' about the various forms of illness but, while sympathetic, they too tend to take for granted the experiential values of pain, dying, disfigurement, fear, anxiety, compulsions and other conditions of the body and mind. All of us may benefit from reflective examination of phenomena of illness and health. Nurses and other healthcare practitioners especially need to be shown, by means of writing, the lived meanings of the phenomena they treat. With such understanding they can be more responsive to people's unique difficulties and more tactful towards people in their communicative relations. And yet, research-as-writing always falls short of its desire to understand the lifeworld. What the listening gaze discerns is not always directly explainable or tellable.

Writing is not just externalising internal knowledge; rather it is the very act of reflective inquiry and of discovery. To research is to write and the insights achieved depend on the right words and phrases, on styles and traditions, on metaphor and figures of speech, on argument and poetic image. Indeed, writing can mean both insight or illusion, living or death. For an author like Derrida (1981) these are values that cannot be decided, fixed or settled since the one always implies, hints at, or complicates the other.

While we do not have to follow Derrida all the way to the certainty of uncertainty, the themes of interpretability and undecidability appear to be helpful. Openness—in the sense of interpretability, undecidability, and tentativeness—is a sustaining motive of phenomenological inquiry. We find it present implicitly and explicitly in the works of phenomenological philosophers. In simple terms it means that we should be modest in claiming special status for our insights. Interpretive phenomenological inquiry is based on the idea that no interpretation is ever complete, no explication of meaning is ever final, no insight is beyond challenge—it behoves us to remain as attentive as possible to life as we live it and to the infinite variety of possible human experiences and possible explications of those experiences. Reading phenomenological texts, if done properly, simulates the process of reflective writing. The reader must write what the author forgot, overlooked, could not 'see' or 'hear'. This is exactly what the editors, Irena Madjar and Jo Ann Walton, and the authors of the chapters in this book invite you to do. They invite you into this interpretive reflective process while you read their wonderfully insightful texts: to deepen them, to enrich them, to personalise them and to test them against life as you encounter and experience it.

REFERENCES

Derrida, J. 1981 *Dissemination* The Athlone Press, London

Van den Berg, J.H. 1972 *Zien: Begrijpen en Verklaren van de Visuele Waarneming* 3rd edn, Callenbach, Nijkerk

Contents

Contributors

Marian Bland RGON, MA, Nurse Specialist, Services for the Elderly, MidCentral Health, Palmerston North, New Zealand

Norma Chick RN, PhD, Emeritus Professor, Massey University, Palmerston North, New Zealand

Ann O'Loughlin RGON, BA, DipSocSci, Senior Lecturer, Department of Nursing and Midwifery, Auckland Institute of Technology, New Zealand

Payom Euswas RN, PhD, Associate Professor, Faculty of Nursing, Mahidol University, Bangkok, Thailand

Irena Madjar RN, PhD, Professor, Faculty of Nursing, University of Newcastle, New South Wales, Australia

Vicki Parker RN, MN, Lecturer, Faculty of Nursing, University of Newcastle, New South Wales, Australia

Kyung-Rim Shin RN, EdD, Associate Professor, College of Nursing, Ewha Womans University, Seoul, Korea

Max van Manen PhD, Professor, Faculty of Education, University of Alberta, Edmonton, Canada

Jo Ann Walton RN, PhD, Associate Professor, Faculty of Nursing, University of Newcastle, New South Wales, Australia

Acknowledgements

THIS BOOK OWES much to the inspiration, encouragement and written contributions of Max van Manen and all the other writers whose work is presented here. We hope that their trust in our ability to present their work as part of something that started for us as a bright idea, but proved rather more difficult in bringing to life, will be justified. Our special thanks go to our families who missed out on what ought to have been a relaxing summer holiday (and many weekends since then), and to our colleagues who at times wondered if anything would emerge from the piles of discarded paper. Most of all, we wish to express our deep gratitude to Judy Waters, who thought the idea of the book was worth supporting when all we had was an outline, who encouraged us through the initial stages, who checked up on us, reminded us and prodded us, and who, like the best of nurses, managed to see the project through even as we despaired.

IRENA MADJAR & JO ANN WALTON
NEWCASTLE, 27 APRIL 1998

Introduction

THIS IS A book about illness and about nursing practice. It is also about what it is like to contemplate the experiences that clients undergo as they live with, or through, an illness episode or health problem, a challenge each of the authors has faced in researching and writing about his or her special interest area. One of our aims is to demonstrate that through phenomenological thinking it is possible to understand such experiences better, and therefore to act more effectively in our dealings with clients, even when we ourselves have not had that particular experience.

Phenomenological inquiry is not new to nursing. The nursing literature contains a large number of phenomenological studies, and those readers who are familiar with the method will need no direction in locating many excellent examples. Our impression is that most of these examples originate from North America, which is unsurprising given the numbers of nurse researchers in that part of the world, the rich research tradition which has grown there over recent decades, and the outstanding examples set by authors and teachers such as Patricia Benner, Nancy Diekelmann, Patricia Munhall, Carolyn Oiler Boyd, Joan Anderson, Vangie Bergum, and others.

We are also aware, however, that in universities around Australia, New Zealand and East Asia there are many nurses undertaking qualitative research studies. Some of this work is published sooner or later, but much of it is not. As academics we are only too conscious that in this region some enlightening and important research is never put out into the public arena in an easily accessible form. One reason is that the format and length for journal publication does not always suit the reporting of a particular research style. So it can be for phenomenological studies which do not easily lend themselves to the conventional research report styles required by most journals. Another is that the opportunities for publication are fewer for nurses in Australasia than in some other parts of the world, such as the USA, Canada and the UK. And yet another reason is that in this part of the world there is a growing but still underdeveloped tradition of writing as a means of sharing knowledge and as a means of fostering professional growth. We hope that this book will go some way towards changing that tradition, while offering readers a different way of presenting our research than the conventional journal format allows.

The idea for this book was born at a workshop on phenomenology run by Max van Manen in Newcastle, New South Wales, in 1996. As Max talked about the work of his North American students, we began to dream of a way of making public some of the phenomenological studies that have been carried out in Australasia. In putting the book together we approached students and ex-students, colleagues and friends whose work we believed would fit together into a compilation such as we envisaged. We have consciously steered away from the format more typical of academic publications; instead the main thrust of the chapters is on the findings of their respective studies, with only a brief introduction to outline the methods employed in the research. We believe that this approach not only allows the authors more freedom than is available in writing traditional research reports, and consequently more scope for rich description and reflection, but that it also makes the reader's part in the process more enjoyable. Rather than beginning each chapter with a detailed and perhaps repetitive account of the research process, the reader is led straight into the body of the work and into the reflective task which reading entails. As editors we acknowledge that our approach is an unconventional one. Perhaps we might not have been so bold had we been less involved in each of the studies that appear here. But in our opinion the approach works, and each chapter stands up to scrutiny in its own right. In our view, the concentration on phenomenological writing that we have encouraged serves well to illustrate just how powerful, and how transformative for engaged readers, such writing can be.

This is not a book about method. It does not attempt to discuss the 'how' of phenomenological research or to be a book that in any way indicates phenomenology to be a 'better' approach than any other for nursing inquiry. Both of us have used the phenomenological approach in our own research and have supervised students who have employed phenomenology in their graduate studies. We believe it to be a wonderful way of thinking about some kinds of problems in nursing. But it is not the only way to approach nursing inquiry, and it cannot be used to answer many important nursing research questions. The studies in this book will, we hope, show just how useful and relevant phenomenology is to nursing, yet we hasten to make it clear that in promoting phenomenological inquiry we do not wish to disparage any other approach that is relevant for finding answers to certain kinds of questions.

The chapters cover a wide range of clinical fields and the authors write about their subjects in different ways. Our aim has been to let readers gain some insight into the work of nurse researchers with a variety of interests, to demonstrate a range of phenomenological writing styles and to encourage readers to think about the impact that reading phenomenology might have on their practice. Readers may detect some influences common to several of the authors' works. Max van Manen's name, in particular, is mentioned repeatedly—his easily accessible writing style and his personal influence on nursing scholarship in Australasia have indeed been significant. Nancy Diekelmann and Patricia Benner have also had significant impact on nursing in this region. Less easy for us to judge is the impact that local scholars—Norma Chick, Jocalyn Lawler, Judith Lumby, Judith Parker, Alan Pearson and others—through their teaching and work with graduate students, have had in bringing phenomenological research into the mainstream in New Zealand, and in adding to its impact in Australia.

The book is organised in two sections. In the first two chapters we present two different perspectives, ours and van Manen's, on the relevance of phenomenology for nursing. Our discussion concentrates on the usefulness of phenomenology as a way of thinking about nursing and the experience of illness and distress that accompanies it. Van Manen's chapter takes a very different approach to the same theme. He shows the reader the importance of different forms of knowledge for nursing practice, and in doing so demonstrates the power of both phenomenological understanding and phenomenological writing. He also offers us new language—the ideas of 'gnostic' and 'pathic' knowing—with which to reflect on the practice of nursing. The remainder of the chapters are derived from individual studies into aspects of illness or nursing practice. They deal with leg ulcers, the experience of intensive care, life with chronic pain, schizophrenic illness, mastectomy, how nurses deal with having to inflict pain while providing care, and what it means for nurses and clients to experience a moment of genuine caring. They also tell of what it feels like to live with a wayward body subjected to hegemonic treatment regimens, what it is like to confront one's own proximity to death, and of the confusion and puzzlement of life on the edge, where technology is at once reassuring and baffling, and where human connection feels lifesaving. They show the intricate connections we experience between mind and body, wherever an illness is located ostensibly and conventionally in diagnostic and commonsense understanding. They describe how nurses contend with pain and suffering which can threaten to overwhelm both them and those for whom they care, and how precious the moments of genuine mutual understanding can be both for clients and nurses.

We believe the book will be of interest to practising nurses, nursing students at undergraduate and graduate level, teachers of nursing and, because of its presentation of a range of writing styles in phenomenology, students of the phenomenological research method in a broader context. We hope readers will enjoy not only the content of each chapter, but also the individual voices of the authors and the context and cultural background reflected in the language in which each author speaks. We believe that studies such as those featured in this book have the potential to increase understanding and so to change attitudes and eventually outcomes of nursing practice. If readers are moved by what they read then we have achieved our major aim.

one

Phenomenology and nursing

JO ANN WALTON & IRENA MADJAR

IT IS NOT easy to define nursing. Nurse theorists and others have tried for several decades now, but while many definitions hold temporary or partial appeal, there is no universally accepted definition. There is something about nursing that defies tidy ordering into boxes, boxes that might be labelled 'scientific', 'technical', 'interpersonal', 'conceptual' or 'clinical'. As nurses know only too well, articulating the essential components of nursing or, more to the point, the whole that is nursing, has become more rather than less difficult.

Yet, curiously, while a definition remains elusive, there is something about the work of nursing that nurses everywhere recognise. When all is said and done, we know that at its best nursing is vitally important in the difference it makes to people who are ill, in pain and in need of care and understanding. Writing about her experiences of nursing in war zones, Etherington (1995, p. 16) states that 'nurses bring a dimension of care to suffering people like no other professionals. Some may ask "what does that mean?" Nurses, however, rarely ask. They already know.'

In this chapter we will explore something of this dimension of care that nurses bring to suffering people. We will discuss the relationships we see between nursing practice, phenomenological research and phenomenological thinking. We hope to show how phenomenology can help us grasp the ordinary, the unexpected and the ineffable elements of human experience in health and illness, and so explain the current interest in phenomenology among members of the nursing discipline. Our intent is to show how and why phenomenology is a relevant and useful form of inquiry for nursing, and we suggest that it has something to do with what it is that nurses 'already know' about nursing.

In her book *Central Mischief*, writer Elizabeth Jolley (1992, p. 51) observes:

> I have been a writer for a longer time than I was a nurse, though it is often said 'once a nurse always a nurse'. There is a connection between nursing and writing. Both require a gaze which is searching and undisturbedly compassionate and yet detached.

This brief observation contains a number of thoughts that bear closer scrutiny. To gaze is 'to look long and fixedly, especially in wonder' (*Collins Concise Dictionary* 1989). What is the purpose of the nursing gaze? Is it a routine part of nursing practice? Is it a skill that can be taught or cultivated? How does a nurse remain detached yet searching and undisturbedly compassionate? Do nurses choose words to describe what they see in the same way that writers do?

Those of us who are familiar with the demands of phenomenological writing may find Jolley's reflection strangely comforting. It is good to know that someone who understands the craft of writing also understands how carefully the nurse looks. Those familiar with the world of clinical practice may be impressed with how simply the writer has captured the complex nature of nursing involvement in clinical situations, including the professional mandate to care and to be prepared to act. Perhaps her acknowledged distance from the world of nursing practice has enhanced Jolley's perception of her previous life and that of her fellow nurses. Certainly her words are richer, deeper and more descriptive than had she referred to 'nursing assessment', a phrase that we are much more likely to hear today than the beautifully crafted sentence quoted above. With the skill of a gifted writer, Jolley has taken a relatively ordinary idea—that there is something similar in the way nurses and writers watch what is going on around them—and has made it into something which stands out in a way that is far from ordinary. To make things stand out in new ways is the challenge of phenomenology. It is also the reward that phenomenology offers.

In many ways Jolley's words cut succinctly to the heart of much of what we wish to say about the relevance of phenomenology for nursing. Phenomenological thinking is not difficult for nurses to grasp since nurses are, as Jolley suggests, accustomed to scanning their horizons for the familiar and the unexpected, using what they see to decide or adjust their actions. They do so with others in mind, as nurses tend to be concerned with others' wellbeing. But they also take things to heart—it is not possible to deal with the intimacy and the out-of-the-ordinary that nursing so often entails without also looking inward.

Phenomenology offers nurses a way of thinking about their practice that is at once simple and familiar, and yet which brings forth understandings that are often novel and complex. The understandings made possible through phenomenological inquiry help to put meaning into the everyday world of practice and of human interaction. Given that nursing is concerned with some of the most intimate occasions in human life, it does not seem surprising that phenomenology, which allows nurses to reflect on the meaning of their work, should be attractive to clinicians and researchers alike. It offers a way to the soul of nursing.

PHENOMENOLOGY AND PHENOMENOLOGICAL INQUIRY

Put very simply, phenomenology is a way of thinking first described by European philosophers, most notably Edmund Husserl, in the first decades of the twentieth century. Phenomenology was further developed and new ideas presented in the work of Martin Heidegger (1927/1962; 1959), Maurice Merleau-Ponty (1962; 1965), Gabriel Marcel (1960; 1965) and Jean-Paul Sartre (1943/1958), all of whom, as Solomon (1987) suggests, were also influential in the development of existentialism. The distinguishing mark of phenomenology is its primary concern with the nature and meaning of human experience. Merleau-Ponty (1962, p. vii) defines phenomenology as 'a study of essences' which requires the researcher to turn to the facticity of the lived world—the world which precedes knowledge and of which knowledge is an abstraction. At the heart of phenomenology is the aim of insightful understanding and description of the phenomena of human experience (van Manen 1990). To make such understanding and description possible, one is required to get behind the labels, behind social and scientific conceptualisations, and follow Husserl's dictum of returning to things themselves, of apprehending human experience as it is lived in the context in which it occurs and which it helps to shape. In Merleau-Ponty's (1962, p. ix) words:

> To return to things themselves is to return to that world which precedes knowledge, of which knowledge always speaks, and in relation to which every scientific schematization is an abstract and derivative sign-language, as is geography in relation to the countryside in which we have learned beforehand what a forest, a prairie or a river is.

In her critical commentary in *Merleau-Ponty's Phenomenology of Perception*, Langer (1989, p. 149) suggests that Merleau-Ponty's central concern 'is to prompt us to recognise that objective thought fundamentally distorts the phenomena of our lived experience, thereby estranging us from our own selves, the world in which we live and other people with whom we interact'. This point is of particular relevance to nursing and nursing inquiry, where so much of what is important in the patient's experience and in the nurse–patient relationship resists objectification and demands understanding and action informed by personal and contextual awareness.

What phenomenology offers is the possibility of studying human experience in the context of the lifeworld. This context includes not only the physical and social environment but also one's history, concerns and aspirations. It is here that meanings are developed and shared. Phenomenological inquiry is therefore able to take into account not only individual meanings of a situation, but also, and more importantly, the intersubjectivity of human experience, the shared meanings that act as a basis for social interaction (Wuthnow et al. 1984).

Perhaps one of the reasons why phenomenology holds such appeal for nurses is its attempt to overcome traditional mind–body dualism through the ideas of 'bodily consciousness' or the 'lived body', developed in particular by Merleau-Ponty (1962) and Marcel (1960; 1965). The body is our basic mode of being in the world, consciousness is embodied consciousness, and a person is embodied being, not just the possessor of a body. In their concern for the whole person, nurses are attracted to the view of the person as embodied spirit—individual and unique but also constrained. The lived, phenomenal body is more than a physical entity. It remembers past hurts, falls ill, smells, hurts, fails to knit together or resists being propelled into the world. It is the phenomenal body, 'the body aware of itself' (Benner & Wrubel 1989, p. 75), that is a means, our only means, of being in the world. The body is the vehicle of our coping and our action in situations where its 'taken-for-grantedness falters' (Kesselring 1990) and discomfort, pain, breathlessness, tiredness or other symptoms become part of the lived experience.

The fit of phenomenology with many questions that interest nurses, and with the person-centred, contextual approach that nursing entails, is now well accepted in the discipline. Examples of published research using a phenomenological approach are too numerous to list. As Munhall (1989) observes, phenomenology emphasises the centrality of subjective reality in human experience and offers a method by which nurses can investigate concerns that are neither simply material, nor easily observable and measurable. The chapters in this volume all provide examples.

THE PLACE OF NARRATIVE IN NURSING

In ordinary conversations, when people attempt to relate something meaningful, to tease out a worry that is bothering them, or to describe their experience of becoming ill or being afraid or ashamed, they often stumble over where to begin, wobble about in the telling, and pause to elaborate at various points along the way. Listening to a story such as this can be difficult. Sometimes it is hard to decide what the point of the story is, or to understand where we are headed, let alone when we will get there. Most of us will ourselves have had the experience of being interrupted while attempting to tell someone about something of importance to us, and will have felt frustrated if the listener wants to hurry us along, to skip the details and get to the point. It can be a challenge to 'get the point' of someone else's story. In our own narratives, the details are necessary if the story is to be told accurately and if we are to feel satisfied that we have conveyed it in its complexity.

In the professional lives of nurses things are often different. In practice situations, one of the greatest challenges and one of the greatest satisfactions of nursing is the quest to get to know the people for whom we care. Nurses pride themselves on their ability to form relationships with their clients, and on the knowledge that stems from these relationships. Even when interventions are brief as, for example, in an emergency department or in day-surgery situations, nurses do their best to get to know something of the clients with whom they are dealing. In any clinical situation, talking and listening to clients and their families is a component of nurses' work. There, nurses are often more prepared than in their 'civilian' lives to hear stories delivered in short segments, or to spend time listening as a story ducks and dives and weaves about, putting the pieces together to form a growing whole.

Nursing entails a special way of observing and listening, and of being present to patients for whom nurses care. It requires attentiveness to individual experiences and to particular situations. Nurses' involvement in the lives of others means that they, as nurses, not only listen to but also tell stories constantly. Over coffee, in hospital corridors, when teaching students, or explaining or defending their practice, nurses tell stories of their work and the people with whom they work. Nursing's oral tradition has helped create a nursing lore from which to draw lessons about nursing, people and life. As Benner, Tanner and Chesla (1996) have pointed out, the practice of storytelling is central to experiential learning and development of clinical expertise. 'The oral tradition is effective in setting up salient memories. Stories are more memorable than lists of warnings that must be memorized out of context.' (1996, p. 208) Nurses learn from their own and from others' experiences and they remember important lessons through stories they tell and hear others tell.

Phenomenology challenges us to go further, and provides a means by which we can. The discipline of the approach requires that the inquiry is systematic, reflective and consensually validated. Yet it starts with an exploration of the individual and the subjective—the experience as it is for the person living it rather than as diagnostic labels might lead us to expect. Nurses have long been presented as being concerned with people as whole persons with individual needs (e.g. Roy 1984; Styles 1982; Travelbee 1971; Watson 1990). At the same time, 'diagnostic related categories' and 'critical pathways' impose expectations on whole categories of patients in terms of their needs, the care they should receive and the patterns of recovery they can be expected to follow. In this context the voice of the individual patient may go unheard, the subjective experience by-passed and the person in need overlooked (Scarry 1985).

Patricia Munhall (1993, p. 125) suggests that to 'be authentically present to a patient' we need to take an open stance and recognise that we do not know the other person and his or her subjective world. Assuming that we know something, or someone, gives us confidence to act. Yet our actions may be quite inappropriate if they are based on what we *presume* to know about the patients in our care rather than on what we have allowed them to teach us about their experience and their need.

Phenomenological accounts of lived experiences of illness present the subjective, the personal, the authentic—experiences from the inside. In doing so they offer a counterpoint to what Audre Lorde in her 'Cancer Journals' identifies as 'that language which has been made to work against us . . . medical language [that] with its "general unifying view" homogenizes [patients'] experience' (cited in Frank 1995, p. 64). Medical language is not always so dehumanising, nor the only one that relies on diagnostic labels to sort people and their needs into manageable categories. Nursing too has its formal and informal ways of simplifying the complexities of human experience by attaching to it names which form part of the 'shorthand' of nursing communication. Such language conceals the complex and sometimes untidy reality of human experience of illness and encourages clinicians to see order where in fact there is disorder.

In exploring the kinds of illness narratives that people tell, Arthur Frank (1995, p. 109) asks that we recognise not only stories of courage and quest for meaning, but that we also 'honour the chaos narrative'—stories of confusion, futility, helplessness and lack of coherence. He asks that we listen to accounts of experiences and emotions for which we may have no remedies. To deny patients a listening ear, the opportunity to communicate their confusion and lostness, is to deny them the dignity of being human. As Frank (1995, p. 112) comments:

> Clinical caregivers steer patients toward medical versions of liberation: treatment plans, rehabilitation, functional normality, lifestyle counseling, remission. These phrases and the many others like them reinstitute the restitution narrative. My objective is hardly to romanticize chaos; it is horrible. But modernity has a hard time accepting, even provisionally, that life sometimes *is* horrible. The attendant denial of chaos only makes its horror worse.

There is a risk that expressions of chaos will be labelled (as anger, denial, depression, or some other 'comprehensible' diagnosis) and once labelled, treated (with drugs or therapy). Such interventions are appropriate in some instances, but in others they deny both the reality of the patient's experience and the possibility of a personal resolution.

When we truly listen, we create a supportive space within which patients can start to make sense of their world. Listening in an engaged and empathetic way to whatever individual patients feel they need to tell us is a means by which nurses show care and provide emotional support. It is an important way by which nurses 'make a difference' to patient outcomes (Benner & Wrubel 1989). But when we truly listen we do something else as well. We compile pictures of individual people and their progress through illness or other experiences, as well as building up our own mental composites of cases. We ponder on the nature of a particular illness or predicament and, as a result, formulate what Benner (1984) and Polanyi (1958) before her have called 'maxims' for practice. Maxims are instructions for action which are developed through repeated exposure to similar situations and reflections on common patterns identified in these situations, and which serve as pointers for future practice.

As professionals, nurses are interested in individual stories but also in the phenomena of human experience. The individual experiences of clients and families are the stuff with which we work. But so are anguish, hope, death, recovery, tragedy, joy and a host of other human conditions. Our professional interest transcends individual experience, or at least does not stop there, because while we attend clinically to individual cases, we must also be able to take our understanding and use it to explore phenomena on a broader basis. That is what learning from experience is about.

Phenomenological inquiry aims to bridge the gap between stories of individual experience and the phenomena of human existence. In this way it speaks to nurses who are familiar with this kind of thinking in their everyday practice situations. Phenomenology can help teach us what we did not know, help us see patterns in the human predicament, and help us develop our practice wisdom.

> Wisdom has nothing to do with the gathering or organizing of facts—this is basic. Wisdom is a seeing through facts, a penetration to the underlying laws and patterns . . . It is one thing to absorb a fact, to situate it alongside other facts in a configuration, and quite another to contemplate that fact at leisure, allowing it to declare its connection with other facts, its thematic destiny, its resonance. (Birkerts 1994, p. 75)

UNNAMING AND UNKNOWING AS ASPECTS OF INQUIRY IN NURSING

As a research method, phenomenology entails a questioning of assumptions, an attempt to go back before conceptual schemas and theoretical explanations, to return to the things themselves. The aim is to present an account of some-thing, some phenomenon, some aspect of human experience, which reveals the phenomenon in question in a new light, one that makes it stand out from the background, enabling us to grasp it in a new way. Often the phenomena, the things with which we are concerned, are common, ordinary, everyday occurrences. At least they are to us as researchers, and in our case, as nurses.

Nurses see aspects of illness, trauma and suffering, or boredom, or pain, or birth, or approaching death almost every day. Each of these things has a name of some kind by which we discuss it with our colleagues and with our clients. There is a shorthand, a series of symbols, a way of representing these phenomena that we expect others to understand. Although we know that these human experiences are filled with emotional, relational, meaningful significance, we do not attend routinely to all these aspects in the everyday. Phenomenology is a way of thinking that allows us to get behind the shorthand, to reveal the experience as it is when it is lived through. Phenomenological thinking is a way of working towards seeing that which is essentially there but which labels and symbols often keep hidden.

To say, for example, that undergoing a femoral artery puncture in order to provide a blood sample 'hurts' is to label the experience in a predictable way that gives it a name but a name that tells us little. It is quite different to be told by a patient that hospital staff 'fish around there, and I say "fish" literally. It should be "harpooning" because if they don't get the [blood] straight away they just keep jabbing and poking . . . The last one took twenty minutes and you just have to lie there as though it isn't happening to you.' (Madjar 1991, p. 160) This patient's description does not name the experience as 'pain' or 'hurt'. What it does is to speak of the embodied and deeply felt experience, inviting us to enter that experience by picturing the weapon and the wounding involved which cannot but be painful.

Described in this way, the phenomenon of clinically inflicted pain can be seen to be different from other pain phenomena—the pain of angina or acute appendicitis or a leg ulcer. The essential painfulness is common to all pain phenomena, but the genesis is different, as is the nature of the experience and the context in which the pain arises and is endured or relieved. Such an understanding of common events in clinical practice can provide nurses with a means of reflecting on how they act in situations in which painful procedures are performed, whatever the context or the procedure.

Much of what nurses do is aimed at giving comfort, relieving symptoms, providing support and information, and making 'faceable' the unknown and the frightening. In doing our work, we often assume that we 'know' what patients are experiencing, or what they need in order to feel comforted, supported or cared for. The assumptions do not have to be wrong—sometimes they involve sound clinical judgement—but they are assumptions nevertheless. To 'really' know, it is necessary sometimes to do what Patricia Munhall (1993, p. 125) suggests: 'stand in one's own socially constructed world and unearth the other's world by admitting, "I don't know your subjective world." . . . In other words, it is essential that we understand our self and our patient to be two distinctive beings, one of whom we do not know.' Such 'unknowing', and the openness needed to make it possible, offers fresh possibilities for knowledge that is true to individual experience. Holding off from naming things, calling into question taken-for-granted assumptions and adopting an open, 'unknowing' stance, are strategies that make phenomenological inquiry exciting. The knowledge arising from such inquiry offers fresh understandings that can inform nursing practice and make it more attuned to patients' needs.

THE LISTENING GAZE

At the beginning of this chapter we discussed Elizabeth Jolley's proposal that nurses and writers have in common a searching gaze—an 'undisturbedly compassionate and yet detached' gaze. Others have written of the medical perspective as a 'clinical gaze [which] has the paradoxical ability to *hear a language* as soon as it *perceives a spectacle*' (Foucault 1963/1975, p. 108). Foucault says that the clinical gaze is an observing gaze that tries to transform what it sees into language, a language that can then be used to teach others lacking the ability to see what is before them, or to see it clearly or adequately. The gaze tends to focus on the manifestations of disease, the unusual and the out-of-the-ordinary, in order to relate these to generalisable patterns conforming to recognised categories of disease (and their diagnostic labels).

The phenomenological gaze, while it tends to focus on the ordinary, may lead to understandings that are extraordinary. Munhall (1994, p. 4) suggests that:

> It is the taken-for-grantedness, the sailing-through-life without reflection, the dazed going-through-the-motions learned from whatever context that give way too often to the meaninglessness and alienation so characteristic of our situated context in the modern age. Phenomenology, as a way of being, takes us from this dazed perspective to a gazed perspective where we give, reflect, and attempt to understand the 'whatness' of everyday life.

Like Jolley's 'gaze which is searching', Munhall uses the term 'gazed perspective' in relation to the phenomenological way of being in the world. In the same way that we commonly say 'I see' when we mean 'I understand', metaphors of vision are common in phenomenological literature. For instance, van Manen (1990, p. 79) says:

> Making something of a text or of a lived experience by interpreting its meaning is more accurately a process of insightful invention, discovery or disclosure—grasping and formulating a thematic understanding is not a rule-bound process but a free act of 'seeing' meaning.

Sartre (1943/1958), on the other hand, when writing about 'the look', reminds us that looking and being the object of someone else's look are not one and the same. To know that I am seen, that someone's gaze is upon me, is not so much to be aware of the person looking but to be made conscious of feeling vulnerable and exposed. In Sartre's words: 'What I apprehend immediately when I hear the branches crackling behind me is not that *there is someone there*; it is that I am vulnerable, that I have a body which can be hurt . . . in short, that *I am seen*.' (Sartre 1943/1958, p. 259)

In nursing, for the most part, we gaze rather than being gazed upon. (The exploration of the patient's experience of being subjected to another's gaze calls for a discussion that lies outside the domain of this book, but it raises issues worth bearing in mind.) Watching, observing, taking note of, attending—these are all actions nurses know well. Yet not all types of watching or looking are socially acceptable. People may also peer, sneak a look, gawp or stare. As nurses we would like to think that the nursing gaze is a positive one, perhaps because of the moral stance that underpins it. Nurses look in the act of caring. In his book *Care of the Soul* Thomas Moore (1992, p. 10) says:

> The basic intention in any caring, physical or psychological, is to alleviate suffering. But in relation to the symptom itself, observance means first of all listening and looking carefully at what is being revealed in the suffering. An intent to heal can get in the way of seeing. By doing less, more is accomplished.

The detached yet compassionate gaze to which Elizabeth Jolley referred and to which Thomas Moore alludes is an important component of phenomenological research. It demands doing less, and it both requires and provokes thought. Van Manen (1983, pp. i–ii) suggests that thoughtfulness is the word that most aptly characterises phenomenology itself:

> To be full of thought means not that we have a whole lot on our mind but rather that we recognize our lot in minding the Whole: that which gives life its fullness. In the works of the great phenomenologists, thoughtfulness is described as a minding, a heeding, a caring attunement—a heedful preoccupation with the project of life, of living, of what it means to live a life.

By stopping to see what is happening we are able to better understand a given phenomenon. We can in some way strip it of its apparent and obvious meanings, digging deeper to find out what is underneath. We try to see through what is presented to us, in an attempt to arrive at a deeper consciousness. As Birkerts (1994, p. 74) points out, we are often embarrassed by terms such as '*truth, meaning, soul, destiny*', but we also hunger for more soul in our work, and we feel better when we are in touch with the depth of it.

The listening gaze that nurses employ is not just a looking gaze. It is a particular stance in the world—an attitude and an openness to others. It is a gaze that is attuned to the concerns of patients and that can adopt different perspectives in order to understand another's experience and to act with care. It is a gaze that is learned through practice and thoughtful and critical reflection. It is such a gaze that allows a nurse to hear the sound of a patient coughing and recognise not only the nature of the cough (moist, dry, raspy, hacking), but also the tiredness of the person exhausted by the effort. Faced with a situation needing intervention, the nurse grasps it as a whole and attends to it with care born of professional attunement.

READING PHENOMENOLOGY

It is one thing to understand what is meant by phenomenological thinking and to recognise how useful this kind of thinking can be in practice; it is another to undertake phenomenological research, and yet another to read phenomenological writing. When phenomenological writing speaks to us, when we recognise and are moved by a phenomenological description, it is first because we understand the situation the author presents to us and, second, because we are helped to understand it differently. All understanding rests on the prior understanding that we have about the thing in question. In order to grasp something we must have a mental picture of it. We must be able to see where and how to take hold of it as an idea. This mental act is dependent on a number of things. It rests on our prior knowledge and understanding of the thing in question, on 'the taste or mood' in our own experiences (Todres 1998), and on our own 'representational processes and desires' (Adams 1986, p. 5). In reading a report of a phenomenological study which deals with some aspect of health, illness or nursing practice we already have a head start.

Suppose we read a study about the experience of pain. Whatever the setting of the particular study, as nurses we have experience of interactions with clients in pain. We have worried about causing pain and about how to relieve it, and we know something of our own reactions towards other people's expressions of pain. We know a range of physical signs that might indicate someone is in pain, and we can think of a great number of circumstances—illnesses, injuries and treatments—that involve pain. We have a repertoire of experiences in which we have helped someone in pain, and also experiences of occasions when an action did not help ease the pain. And as human beings each of us knows some other things about pain. We know what our own pain feels like, whether in toothache, migraine or fracture, or in childbirth or after surgery. We know what helps and what doesn't when we are in pain, and that others do not respond in quite the same way. We also know that no-one else feels our pain. If they did they would not offer some of the remedies they try. In addition, we know that grief hurts, so pain is not always a result of a physical cause. All of these ideas are with us as we read. They form the background on which the writer's words will fall.

Whatever way the data are collected, and from whatever source, the phenomenological researcher must engage in writing and rewriting in order that a phenomenological description is produced (van Manen 1990). Because the writing process is so central, it is in some ways essential to practise phenomenological writing in order to understand it. Or, as Solomon (1987, p. 161) has put it, 'one is rightly warned by practicing phenomenologists that one needs to develop a taste for phenomenology and some feeling for its workings before one can be in a position to say what it is'. All writing requires an audience if the understandings contained within it are to be made public and open to scrutiny and validation.

But the process of reading a phenomenological study can also have an effect on the reader. Birkerts (1994, p. 80) writes about this effect of reading on the reader, suggesting that reading is an act that can transport us, that can result in a major 'internal transition', a change of mental state. He reflects also on the initial act of engagement with a text. In choosing what to read we exhibit a degree of willingness, of openness to discovery and new perspectives and insights. Our prior understanding (even if this is just an understanding of how little we know) leads us to wanting to explore further.

Reading is about understanding, about getting hold of ideas and having them mean something to us personally. Dilthey (1926/1994) suggests that the act of reading involves an empathetic state of mind and a certain readiness within readers to consider the text before them. Like poetry, which Dilthey (1926/1994, p. 159) uses in his discussion of understanding, phenomenological writing can engage the reader on a deep, personal level:

> The approach of higher understanding to its object is determined by its task of discovering a vital connection in what is given. This is only possible if the context which exists in one's own experience and has been encountered in innumerable cases is always—and with all the potentialities contained in it—present and ready . . . Potentialities of the soul are evoked by the comprehension—by means of elementary understanding—of physically presented words. The soul follows the accustomed paths in which it enjoyed and suffered, desired and acted in similar situations. Innumerable roads are open, leading to the past and dreams of the future; innumerable lines of thought emerge from reading.

The internal transition that results from reading phenomenology is twofold. On the one hand, the reader is drawn into the project of making the phenomenon under discussion understandable and taking it out of the private arena and into the public. Reinharz (1983) describes this as a series of epistemological transformations that begin when the person living the experience uses language and actions to communicate the experience to a researcher. The researcher in turn must transform this communication into a personal understanding of the described experience, and then into concepts that capture the essential qualities of the original experience. The ideas and concepts are then crafted into a written document, a paper, a dissertation, a book chapter which is then presented to an audience. It is the audience that provides the final transformation by relating the ideas to their experience, clarifying their past understandings and (hopefully) 'seeing' things in a new light. Good phenomenological writing aided by anecdotes and stories that ground the interpretations in the reality of lived experience, has the capacity to exert a powerful influence. In this sense, phenomenological writing can engage and inspire our imaginations in ways that facts and figures seldom do.

On the other hand, the main practical benefit of phenomenology is one that is not easily seen. It tells us of the 'depth' of an experience and the nature of the phenomenon, but not the extent or prevalence of the problem. Phenomenological research does not offer technical solutions or answers. Instead, the benefits of phenomenological inquiry are to be found 'in the reform of understanding, in what its serious pursuit "does with us"'(Burch 1989, p. 204). This effect is one we ourselves feel. It encourages in us the possibility of more thoughtful actions and wiser conduct (Burch 1989).

The moral dimension of nursing is well recognised and has been written about extensively (Bishop 1996; Bishop & Scudder 1990, 1991; Watson 1985). Indeed, Watson (1985), Benner and Wrubel (1989) and other nurse scholars, stress the primacy of personal engagement and moral concern for nursing practice. Other writers have made similar comments about other helping professions. Dokecki (1996), for example, identifies trustworthiness, prudence and caring as central virtues for those engaged in human helping professions.

Phenomenology offers nurses and other human helpers a way of thinking about their practice realm and the recipients of their care, a ground from which to act more thoughtfully, tactfully and carefully. It also offers a way of restructuring our reflections on our work more wisely and more usefully. As research, phenomenological inquiry draws on precisely this kind of reflectiveness. It entails attentiveness to individual experience and the ability to shed fresh light on the shared human condition through careful analysis and writing. The end product, a report of the phenomenological study, is still one step from completion. It is in the understanding and consequent actions of the reader that the study finally impacts on practice. We hope that some of the studies in this book will inspire, challenge and change your understanding of some aspect of your practice world.

REFERENCES

Adams, J. 1986 *The Conspiracy of the Text: The Place of Narrative in the Development of Thought* Routledge & Kegan Paul, London

Benner, P. 1984 *From Novice to Expert: Excellence and Power in Clinical Nursing Practice* Addison-Wesley, Menlo Park, Ca.

Benner, P., Tanner, C.A. & Chesla, C.A. 1996 *Expertise in Nursing Practice: Caring, Clinical Judgment, and Ethics* Springer Publishing Company, New York

Benner, P. & Wrubel, J. 1989 *The Primacy of Caring: Stress and Coping in Health and Illness* Addison-Wesley, Menlo Park, Ca.

Birkerts, S. 1994 *The Gutenberg Elegies* Faber and Faber, London

Bishop, A. 1996 'The nature of nursing' in *Truth in Nursing Inquiry* eds J.F. Kikuchi, H. Simmons & D. Romyn, Sage, Thousand Oaks, Ca.

Bishop, A. & Scudder, J.R. Jr 1990 *The Practical, Moral and Personal Sense of Nursing: A Phenomenological Philosophy of Practice* State University of New York Press, Albany

——1991 *Nursing: The Practice of Caring* National League for Nursing, New York

Burch, R. 1989 'On phenomenology and its practices' *Phenomenology + Pedagogy* vol. 7, pp. 187–217

Collins Concise Dictionary 1989 William Collins Sons & Co., London & Glasgow

Dilthey, W. 1926/1994 'The hermeneutics of the human sciences' *The Hermeneutics Reader* ed. K. Mueller-Vollmer, Continuum, New York

Dokecki, P. 1996 *The Tragi-Comic Professional: Basic Considerations for Ethical Reflective-Generative Practice* Duquesne University Press, Pittsburgh, Pa.

Etherington, C. 1995 'Working in international war zones: A personal account' *Tennessee Nurse* vol. 58, no. 5, pp. 14–16

Foucault, M. 1963/1975 *The Birth of the Clinic: An Archeology of Medical Perception* (trans. A.M. Sheridan Smith) Vintage Books, New York

Frank, A.W. 1995 *The Wounded Storyteller: Body, Illness, and Ethics* The University of Chicago Press, Chicago and London

Heidegger, M. 1927/1962 *Being and Time* (trans. J. Macquarrie & E. Robinson) Basil Blackwell, Oxford

——1959 *An Introduction to Metaphysics* (trans. R. Manheim) Yale University Press, New Haven

Jolley, E. 1992 *Central Mischief* Viking Books, Ringwood, Victoria

Kesselring, A. 1990 *The Experienced Body, When Taken-for-Grantedness Falters: A Phenomenological Study of Living with Breast Cancer* unpublished PhD thesis, University of California, San Francisco

Langer, M.M. 1989 *Merleau-Ponty's Phenomenology of Perception: A Guide and Commentary* Macmillan Press, London

Madjar, I. 1991 *Pain as Embodied Experience: A Phenomenological Study of Clinically Inflicted Pain in Adult Patients* unpublished PhD thesis, Massey University, Palmerston North

Marcel, G. 1960 *Mystery of Being* Henry Regnery Co. (Gateway edition), Chicago

——1965 *Being and Having* Collins (Fontana edition), London

Merleau-Ponty, M. 1962 *Phenomenology of Perception* (trans. C. Smith), Routledge & Kegan Paul, New York

——1965 *The Structure of Behaviour* (trans. A.L. Fisher) Methuen, London

Munhall, P.L. 1989 'Philosophical ponderings on qualitative research methods in nursing' *Nursing Science Quarterly* vol. 2, no. 1, pp. 20–8

——1993 '"Unknowing": Toward another pattern of knowing in nursing' *Nursing Outlook* vol. 41, no. 3, pp. 125–8

——1994 *Revisioning Phenomenology: Nursing and Health Science Research*, National League for Nursing Press, New York

Moore, T. 1992 *Care of the Soul: A Guide for Cultivating Depth and Sacredness in Everyday Life* HarperCollins, New York

Polanyi, M. 1958 *Personal Knowledge: Towards a Post-Critical Philosophy* Routledge & Kegan Paul, London

Reinharz, S. 1983 'Phenomenology as a dynamic process' *Phenomenology + Pedagogy* vol. 1, no. 1, pp. 77–9

Roy, C. 1984 *Introduction to Nursing: An Adaptation Model* 2nd edn, Prentice-Hall, Englewood Cliffs, NJ.

Sartre, J. 1943/1958 *Being and Nothingness* (trans. H.E. Barnes) Methuen, London

Scarry, E. 1985 *The Body in Pain* Oxford University Press, New York

Solomon, R.C. 1987 *From Hegel to Existentialism* Oxford University Press, New York

Styles, M.M. 1982 *On Nursing: Toward a New Endowment* C.V. Mosby Company, St Louis, Mi.

Todres, L. 1998 'The qualitative description of human experience: The aesthetic dimension' *Qualitative Health Research* vol. 8, no. 1, pp. 121–7

Travelbee, J. 1971 *Interpersonal Aspects of Nursing* 2nd edn, F.A. Davis Company, Pa.

van Manen, M. 1983 'Invitation to Phenomenology + Pedagogy' (Editorial) *Phenomenology + Pedagogy* vol. 1, no. 1, pp. i–ii.

——1990 *Researching Lived Experience: Human Science for an Action Sensitive Pedagogy* Althouse Press, London & Ontario

Watson, J. 1985 *Nursing: The Philosophy and Science of Caring* Colorado Associated University Press, Boulder, Colorado

——1990 'Transpersonal caring: A transcendent view of person, health, and healing' *Nursing Theories in Practice* ed. M. Parker, National League for Nursing Press, New York

Wuthnow, R., Hunter, J.D., Bergesen, A. & Kurzweil, E. 1984 *Cultural Analysis: The Work of Peter L. Berger, Mary Douglas, Michel Foucault, and Jürgen Habermas* Routledge & Kegan Paul, London *two*

The pathic nature of inquiry and nursing

MAX VAN MANEN

WHEN WE GET to know someone or something really well we sometimes use a special name, a nickname. A nickname is really a name over and above the name that something or someone already carries. The original meaning of sur-name (from the French word *surnom*) implies a renaming, the placement of a second name above or on top (*sur*) the first name.[1] With the nickname we indicate our special relation to something or someone. We make our world knowable by giving names, assigning labels to them. But nicknames and proper names serve a special function. They (re)name the often more subjectively felt meanings of our relations with others.

Giving names is a most peculiar act. What occurs when one *gives* a name?, asks Derrida (1995). What does one give? One does not offer a thing. One delivers nothing. And yet something comes to be. What is this something? And why do we rename? We seem to rename when the usual name is found to be lacking of something. Sometimes ordinary words have become too ordinary; we feel the need to get at what is unique, personal, singular, untranslatable about that which we name.

We could push the problem further, beyond the cognitive towards the unnameable, the pathic dimensions of life. In order to explore the living relations we maintain with the world we first need to unname things. In the short story 'She unnames them' the science fiction author Ursula Le Guin (1987) hints at what happens in unnaming.

Le Guin tells the tale of a woman who asks Adam to take back her name, a name he had given her just as he had given names to all the animals that the Creator had brought before him. First she persuaded the animals and the birds and the insects and the fishes to accept namelessness. They agreed and decided to give back their names. For most of them the act of unnaming was very easy since the names given to them had left them utterly indifferent. The woman must have suspected that the effect of unnaming might be quite dramatic. But the effect she sought, of becoming more attached to the world, was even more powerful than she had anticipated. After the unnaming she discovered with surprise how close she felt to the creatures around her. 'They seemed far closer than when their names had stood between myself and them like a clear barrier: so close that my fear of them and their fear of me became one and the same fear.' (Le Guin 1987, p. 195)

In a strange way, after the unnaming, things became indistinguishable from one another. The desire to smell one another's smells, to feel or rub one another's scales, fur, feathers, or skin was now so immediate and created such sense of presence that she decided that she could make no exception and she too needed to give back the name that had been given to her. So she went up to Adam and said: 'You and your father lent me this—gave it to me, actually. It's been really useful, but it does not exactly seem to fit very well lately. But thanks very much! It's really been very useful.' (Le Guin 1987, p. 196)

She found that it was not that easy to return a gift without creating the impression of being ungrateful. But Adam seemed preoccupied. 'He was not paying much attention, as it happened, and said only, "Put it down over there, OK?" and went on with what he was doing.' (Le Guin 1987, p. 196) After some hesitation she said at last to him, 'Well, goodbye, dear. I hope the garden key turns up.' (p. 196)

With this simple tale Ursula Le Guin produces a scene that is no less startling than the philosophical reflections of Derrida (1995) on the meaning of name. When things get unnamed we can no longer ignore the hidden contours of the phenomena that words tend to hide like blankets of snow. For Adam language was only a tool to gain dominion over the earth and its inhabitants.

> He was fitting parts together, and said without looking around, 'OK, fine dear. When's dinner?'
>
> 'I'm not sure,' I said. 'I'm going now. With the—' I hesitated, and finally said, 'With them, you know,' and went on. In fact I had only just then realized how hard it would have been to explain myself. I could not chatter away as I used to do, taking it all for granted. My words now must be as slow, as new, as single, as tentative as the steps I took going down the path away from the house, between the darkbranched, tall dancers motionless against the winter shining. (Le Guin 1987, p. 196)

Reflecting on words or names helps us to realise how closely related language is to thinking and to our ways of being in the world. But exactly what occurs when we unname things is a question that is rarely asked. Can we truly erase the words we give to the things that are important to us? How would we unname pain, illness, anxiety, nursing or healing?

We do not live in the science-fiction world created by Le Guin. We cannot unname everything, perhaps not even one thing. But unnaming does not have to mean that we completely discard words. By putting words aside or by making them transparent we can orient to our world as if we were removing a 'clear barrier' that stands between us and our lived experiences. Certainly we would not be able to take things for granted as we usually do.

Think how we would have to orient to illness. We could no longer assume, for example, that this or that illness is known by its diagnostic label, that the clinical path of disease is what matters most, that asthma is asthma, that diverticulitis is diverticulitis. We would have to unname the illness and study the complexity, subjectivity and variability of different people's lives. Of course, the purpose of this unnaming exercise would not be to let go of all the progress made in medical science. But to understand people's experience we would need to get really close to them so that their hopes become our hopes, their pain becomes our pain—we would need to listen and speak, read and write in a manner that is attentive to the things of the world that are ultimately unnameable. Our words would now have to be 'as slow, as new, as single, as tentative' as if we were going down a path away from the familiar towards a world we have never navigated before.

Indeed, this is the project of interpretive phenomenological inquiry. By unnaming things we gain the opportunity to explore their pathic or lived dimensions—our 'moods' or ways of being in the world.

PATHIC LANGUAGE FOR PATHIC LIVING

Some things are so much part of the to and fro of living that it is difficult to unname them. Breathing is such an example. What is more common than breathing? On the one hand breathing and its mechanisms for oxygen consumption and carbon dioxide production are well understood. We take part in a continual exchange of air with our environment, and yet most of us rarely think about it. Unless we engage in yoga or suffer from a respiratory illness we tend not to reflect on breathing. On average we inhale and exhale air twenty times a minute, about six- or seven-hundred million breaths in a lifetime. We may take slow and deliberate big gulps of air at the seaside, we may sniff the delicate bouquet of a fine wine, we may huff and puff in exhilaration after strenuous exercise, or we may hold our mouth and nose in disgust at the repulsive odour of a passing diesel engine.

Breathing appears to become a particularly subjective matter when the need for breathing increases. But what is perceived when we breathe? Who (what part of our being) has this experience? Is it the physiological, 'automaton' self, the pathic existence of the ventilating mechanism which, like the self-regulating heartbeat, makes breathing an experience that is rarely noticed? Is breathing mostly a non-experience? Or is it the person himself or herself who breathes? How do we experience this respiratory fact of our existence? Buytendijk (1974, pp. 282, 283) speaks of breathing as a sort of 'being tuned'. But, while he details the physiology of breathing, he also notes that we know few ways to describe the pathic or bodily lived dimension of it.

We sometimes seem to get out of tune with our world. This occurs, for example, in the sigh of exasperation, the heave of relief or the gasp of terror. Breathing becomes the basis for experiences which are representative of moods and feelings. Do we sigh deeply because we are out of tune with our world? If so, in what sense? Words seem to fall short when we try to describe this sense of being out of tune.

Breathing in is not experienced in the same manner as breathing out. They differ in the tensions we feel. Exhaling seems more passive, a relaxing of the muscles towards a moment of rest. Inhaling is the opposite movement where the muscles are tensed. The whole process of breathing seems to be a condition of restlessness, a restlessness that belongs to living, to being alive.

When we hold our breath, or when we cannot breathe for a moment, we immediately become aware of a different mood. We sense a growing desperation. A tension mounts in our chest—we must *do* something to still this hunger, air hunger. Soon panic grips.

'Asthma' is originally a Greek word meaning 'hard-drawn breath'. When Sasha Clarke thinks back to her childhood experience of asthma she remembers it as a struggle with time (Clarke 1997, p. 2):

> I always felt like I was running out of time for some reason. I think maybe it was that I thought I couldn't last a second longer. It was as though my chest was going to cave in on me and I just wasn't going to be able to take enough breaths so that I would last until they could fix me.
>
> I always told my Mum that this was the worst one ever but she always said that it was just the same as last time. I never believed her. I used to think she wouldn't say that if she could crawl inside my body

> right now, but I learned later that she was right. I think it was just because I was so scared. Sometimes I used to cry and that only made it worse, so I stopped.

For Sasha's mother, Monica, asthma visited often in the middle of the night (Clarke 1997, pp. 2, 3). Time is measured by breath; breathlessness turns into a strange sense of timelessness.

> I was asleep when I heard the asthma find a new tempo of assault. Closed doors, but I knew and I was up, the dark house sliding past me. She sits Buddhawise in the middle of her bed, hands on knees, shoulders high and wide, mouthing speechless words. I help her with the inhaler and there is some relief for the words come—'Mummy, Mummy'—a small breathless chant.
>
> I pick her up, her arms around my neck. She grips but holds herself away, straining upward and leaning back with the need to have space all around her chest. We go into the kitchen, all blue shadows in the night light. I put her on a high stool, her arms up on a pillow on the kitchen counter. We try the inhaler again. This is wrong, I know. She has already had too much and it is not working.
>
> Dark curls matted stuck to her forehead, all of her sweaty under my hands. Little shoulders, ribs. Her lips are dark blackish in the dim kitchen light. I have to decide what to do, but I am empty and stupid. My thoughts fly high above the moment, not touching us, not present. I am outside myself watching the scene that unfolds like a bad movie.
>
> We wait in the darkened kitchen for nothing. Time is gone. There are only the two of us in this other world where moments are measured by the flailing labored breathing.
>
> She starts a barking cough so demanding that there is no space for breaths. Her eyes fill to cry and I am there living in my anger and my fear. 'Stop that, don't cry, just breathe damn you, breathe?' I have my car keys, a coat, a blanket. I throw words to the others in the sleeping house. 'We are going to the hospital!'

Medically speaking, asthma is defined as an obstructive disease of the pulmonary airways due to spasms of the smooth muscles within the airways, increased mucous secretion and inflammation. But if we want to understand the experience of asthma closely we must attend to how it presents itself to those who live it. Monica Clarke wrote about her experience of asthma as part of a research seminar. Here we discover that phenomenological research requires a special attentiveness to the pathic side of language. In this instance, for both mother and daughter, asthma is experienced, in part, as time. Running out of air is running out of time. Time becomes measured by every gasping breath. Time becomes breathing. Breathing time. For a small child in the throes of a severe asthma attack every time becomes the one time. Every time becomes the one worst time ever. A crisis point. This crisis point of time becomes a turning point in life, a turning point of life—will there be breath? Will there be time this time? Will there be life after breath? (Clarke 1997).

THE PATHIC NATURE OF PRACTICE

During a recent seminar, Jean van der Zalm, a nurse educator, mentioned several innocent incidents that occurred during her teaching of student nurses.[2] These incidents would have been forgotten quickly if they had not happened that same morning.

During her talk, Jean explained that student nurses must learn to rely on their sense of sight, touch, hearing and smell to detect abnormalities in the physical condition of patients. The techniques used include inspection, palpation, percussion and auscultation. Quite literally the nurse scrutinises very closely and minutely the skin and body of the patient by watching, feeling, sensing, touching, pressing, stroking, vibrating, tapping, blowing, striking, smelling and listening. As we listened to Jean's explanations, the other graduate students (from education and psychology) in our seminar could not help but gain the impression that these practices are, potentially at least, highly charged with the intimacy of human touch.

On the morning of the incidents, Jean had introduced her students to palpation, a technique of physical examination. Most medical texts define palpation as 'the act of feeling by the sense of touch' but this definition is too limited for the complex meanings that a practised hand can extract (DeGowin & DeGowin 1976, p. 35). The human hand is marvellously equipped to be receptive to different types of sensations. Medical and nursing handbooks provide a great deal of detail about the practice of palpation and the sensory discriminations detected through the use of the hand. Because of its anatomical structure the hand possesses regional sensitivities and degrees of receptivity to different types of sensations. The fingerpads are most sensitive to moisture, contour, consistency and mobility; fingertips are especially suited to exploring tiny skin lesions; the dorsal surface and the ulnar edge of the hand and fingers are most sensitive to variations of temperature; the palmar surface, or ball of the hand, best detects vibratory impulses.

Deep palpation refers to the application of firmer pressure to examine the condition of deeper organs and structures. Light palpation is used for detecting skin surface characteristics and structures located immediately below the skin. This type of palpation, using various parts of the hands and fingers, is the most common method for examining a patient's face, neck, axilla, chest, breast, abdomen and extremities. Students must learn to let their fingers glide, roll and gently push across the skin of the patient. A course guide (Kot, n.d., p. 13) describes in a matter-of-fact tone how the hand becomes a data-collecting instrument that is manipulated in a diagnostic manner:

> Maneuvering the position of the palpating hand and varying the type of motion will affect the type of data collected. Gliding the fingerpads over the skin surface in a horizontal and vertical plane will yield data on texture and surface contour. Information about the position and consistency of a structure can be obtained by using the grasping fingers.

Any patient who has been submitted to a palpation examination of a cystic breast or abdominal complaint may recall that this was hardly a pleasant experience. But student nurses who must practise palpation on each other find this experience unpleasant for more ambiguous reasons. Jean described her students' experiences as follows:

> *In a three-hour morning lab I taught the students palpation and I noticed that they seemed to be uncomfortable. First, some students confided in me during the break that they were quite reluctant to have Ken, an only male student nurse in the class, participate in the peer practice. During peer practice one student must put on the patient gown and the other the nursing uniform. Even though Ken has many years of ambulance experience and though he is a very pleasant person, the students felt extremely uneasy having to pair up with Ken and practise palpation. We solved the problem by having Ken practise on a dummy. Some female students even felt uncomfortable doing the palpation on each other and some asked if they could keep on their underwear under the gown.*

Jean explained that, though being undressed in the company of one's peers may be embarrassing, nurses must learn to do palpation. Keeping on underwear is not allowed since it inhibits the process of sensitive discriminations of skin on skin, especially if the underwear is long or elastic.

The second incident happened when the students had to move out of the lab into the ward where they had to apply their palpating techniques to elderly patients. The students kept postponing, lingering and stalling. In Jean's words, they seemed willing to do anything to avoid doing palpations. When Jean finally confronted them, the student nurses admitted that they were quite hesitant. What if these patients did not want to be bothered? What if they were reading or taking a nap? What if they had different things on their minds?

When Jean in her next class asked students to reflect on the nature of their reluctance to practise palpation on each other and on patients they were happy to talk about it. They admitted that their difficulties had to do with ambiguity. They felt acutely aware that there are different ways of touching and that some forms of touching are not fitting for palpation. When asked about these differences students made a spontaneous distinction between what they called professional touching and non-professional touching.

What then is professional touching?, Jean asked. Students responded by saying that 'the professional touch is firm not light, confident and directed with purpose, goal and intent'. One student said: 'When I was practising palpation on my sister at home I was too gentle. She told me not to touch in this way. She said it was too light and might be misinterpreted by the patient.' When Jean asked the students to describe non-professional touching they said, 'It is hard to describe but it is easy to know when it is not right.'

Another incident occurred as the students were practising palpatation on the elderly patients in the ward. A patient was uncooperative and shirked away when one of the student nurses tried to do her palpation examination. The woman seemed so upset that a nurse, who was present, put her hand on the woman's arm in a gesture of support. The patient surrendered to the nurse's hands and started sobbing. 'Isn't it strange,' remarked the nurse later, 'that the patient rejected the hands of one nurse but reached out to the hands of another!' And of course it is somewhat ironic that while the young nurse had tried so earnestly to apply the correct touch, this was not received well by the patient. The irony is that it was not an issue of a professional touch versus a non-professional touch; rather the patient needed not the gnostic touch of palpation but the pathic touch of support.

So it seems that there are at least two kinds of touch that we might distinguish in reflecting on the situation of the nursing students: the gnostic and the pathic touch.

The (dia)gnostic touch

First there is the gnostic touch of palpation as described in medical texts. The objective of palpation is diagnostic. Literally (dia)gnostic means 'to know thoroughly' in the sense of 'seeing through the body'. The palpating hand can bring about this diagnostic 'view'. A medical text (Kot, n.d., p. 9) states that the 'assessment of underlying anatomical structures is facilitated if the examiner makes a habit of mentally visualizing anatomical features while conducting the examination'. Thus we may say that palpation belongs primarily to the gnostic or medical side of healthcare—both doctor and nurse apply the procedure with diagnostic intent. This is how a doctor describes the uncannily effective (dia)gnostic skill of palpation:[3]

> *It was my second week as the intern on ICU. The unit was to receive an admission from the ward momentarily. The previous evening the patient had undergone emergency surgery for a ruptured appendix and was now doing poorly. She presented with fever, tachycardia and tachypnoea; she was definitely septic. I initially focused my exam on the patient's abdomen as this was the site of the surgical incision.*
>
> *Carefully, I removed the dressings and provided reassurance to the patient. I expected this exam to be difficult. On inspection, there was clear fluid oozing out of the incision. It was swollen, red and looked angry. I began my exam with light palpation in the opposite corner and worked my way across the abdomen. I could feel the tenseness in the abdominal muscles, especially the rectus abdominis. Gently, I asked the patient to bring her knees up. I wanted to examine the abdomen with the muscles relaxed. My plan was to examine the surgical incision last, because I knew this would cause her the most pain. Following a normal light palpation, I performed a deeper palpation of the abdomen, attempting to feel for masses. As long as I avoided the surgical site, she tolerated the procedure well.*
>
> *It was time to move to the hot area. As I rolled my fingers lightly over the surgical incision, I had a passing feeling of bubbles, crepitations, in the abdominal wall. I knew this was not benign air in the muscles. Until proved otherwise I had to treat the case as gas gangrene. I immediately called for a swab and requested a stat gram stain to confirm my clinical suspicion. I then continued with the rest of the abdominal exam. Upon deep palpation and rapid removal of the hands, there was marked rebound tenderness, signifying inflammation around the surgical site. I had my answer.*
>
> *Shortly after, the lab confirmed my diagnosis. Now I faced the real problem. I immediately marked the skin to demonstrate the extent of the crepitations and booked the patient for emergency surgery. In the following 24 hours she had three debridement surgeries and thankfully survived.*

In this example of the lifesaving power of the gnostic touch, we sense the close relation between the expert gnostic eye, the gnostic mind and the gnostic touch. While the doctor remains aware of the vulnerability of the patient as a person, his care for her predicament is expressed in a gnostic approach to her suffering.

The term gnostic derives from the Greek word *gnōstikós*, meaning 'one who knows'; the notion is related to mind, judgement, maxim and opinion. In the second century, Gnosticism emerged as the sectarian belief that reason is the proper device by which to teach and practise religion. In its extreme forms, Gnosticism involved the mystical revelation of supernatural knowledge for an elite of knowers and saviours.

In our age, at a more secular level, the gnostic attitude in medicine and the health sciences also proceeds on the principle that the process of healing is approached and defined in terms of rationalistic factors. It is not surprising, therefore, that we find the term 'gnostic' in the most commonly used medical terminology, 'diagnostic' and 'prognostic'. To the layperson, gnostic knowledge may still command an element of awe and blind faith. And yet, as the general public becomes more rationally informed of medical knowledge, the image of the physician as a holy healer seems to be eroding.

The probing gnostic touch

The diagnostic touch can be seen as a specialisation of the more general cognitive and probing aspects of touch. Touch is perhaps the most fundamental feature of human experience, letting us explore, discover and know the world and ourselves in a perceptually unique manner. Touching is finding something tactile. And the hand is uniquely suited to its probing task. The touch of our hand lets us explore the materiality of the world around us. That is why we say that we learn to 'handle' and 'manipulate' things. The phenomenology of touch is quite subtle and complex.

We all know from experience that to touch something and to be touched by something are two very different experiences—even though in both cases the objective pressure on the skin may be exactly the same. When something unexpectedly touches us then we may shrink back. Moreover, when something or someone touches me, I do not only feel the other, I also feel myself. When I suddenly experience the touch of the other person I do not only feel the skin of the other's hand, I also feel myself, through my own skin. This is even true when, for example, my right hand touches my left hand. Merleau-Ponty called this phenomenon a kind of physical reflection (1964, p. 166). He shows how in the handshake I feel the other's hand as if it were my own other. So there is a dual aspect to the touch of things: through touch we get to know what is outside of us; at the same time we become aware of ourselves together with that which is being touched (Merleau-Ponty 1964, pp. 166–72).

So what does this mean for palpation? The patient who is being palpated is in the position of feeling the palpating hand of a nurse or physician and at the same time feeling his or her own body. The probing hand turns anatomical, and it is quite possible that the patient begins to participate in the probing attitude. At least that is how one person describes the experience:

> *As I was lying prone on the hard, narrow examination table, the physician was probing my abdomen. Slightly embarrassed by this procedure, my eye caught the anatomical charts on the wall where an opened-up torso exposed its various organs and muscle groups. While turning my face away from the doctor I fleetingly focused on the intestines in the picture. I was imagining what the hand on my abdomen might be feeling and I was hoping that there would not be any evidence of some villainous lump or malignant growth. I tried not to be tense, but then the sudden push–pull movement of the physician's hands caused excruciating pain.*
>
> *After I had rearranged my clothes the doctor explained that I probably suffered from diverticulitis, an infectious condition of the colon; not uncommon for someone my age. He drew me a picture of diverticular pockets on the colon wall. An X-ray would have to confirm the diagnosis.*
>
> *As I left the doctor's office and walked onto the busy street, I felt a bit unsettled—as if my abdomen had been left exposed somehow. The doctor's hands had given me X-ray eyes. In the street, instead of people, I saw fleshy torsos marching by. Torsos filled with blood, organs, intestines. How would I ever be able to just see people rather than stuffed torsos wrapped in skin and clothes? I had walked into the doctor's office with the simple complaint of a sore stomach but now my diseased colon was in conspiracy with the unappetising anatomies of the people passing me by in the street.*

How many people, as patients, undergo this strange sensation of X-ray eyes? The phenomenologist Van den Berg describes a similar experience as a young medical student in the 1930s in an anatomy lab in the Netherlands. He recalls a moment when he and a female medical student had to practise their anatomical skills on a corpse (1959, p. 220):

> I dissected at that moment the musculature of the shoulder and upper arm, my practicum companion dissected the lower arm and hand . . . When I looked up at what she was doing I perceived two hands: the hand belonging to the corpse and the hand of my fellow student.
>
> The live hand was nicely tanned and slightly manicured. Slightly, because female medical students are not terribly preoccupied with manicure. One only needs to imagine a hand adorned with rings and heavily lacquered with nailpolish holding the knife and scalpel. The difference between the two hands would have been spoiled. But now this strange difference presented itself. Two hands. Under the moving, easily manipulating hand of the living lay the hand of the dead. A parched, white, withered, dried-up hand. A dead hand. A pathetic hand. A split open, busted, jammed open, gaping hand. A terrible hand. A hand with muscles, tendons, veins, nerves, membranes, bands and bones. A full, stuffed, filled hand. A belabored hand. A fussed over hand.
>
> And above it, active, mobile, moving, a simple hand, a closed hand of the young woman. Only a slight sign, some blue veins on its back.

Van den Berg (1959) argues that around the year 1300 a significant event in human history occurred, when the ordinary closed body was first cut open and anatomised by Mundinus and later by others. From this moment onwards it is possible to see the hand with two kinds of vision: with the gnostic eye and with the pathic eye. We can even see this gnostic eye portrayed in Rembrandt's paintings of anatomy lessons.

But, like the analytical eye, the hand itself has become gnostic. The two hands that Van den Berg saw—one alive and dissecting, the other dead and anatomised—both belong to the gnostic domain. And yet he could not help but also see a different hand—the closed and natural looking hand of his fellow student. This is the pathic hand, the pathic body, which remains resistant to X-ray eyes. Van den Berg saw a 'nicely tanned and slightly manicured' hand touching an anatomised hand which was being dissected in a gnostic manner. The pathic hand belonged to the female student beside him. But, at the same time, her hand was performing a gnostic task. Thus, Van den Berg saw the hands even more ambiguously than he himself describes: both as gnostic and as pathic.

The private pathic touch

The pathic touch is no less complex than the gnostic touch—it too may be experienced in a variety of modalities. Within the context of the discussion on palpation, it is possible to distinguish between a private and a personal touch, though these too have several experiential dimensions. The private touch may be loving, friendly, erotic or intimate; the personal touch may be experienced as supportive, caring, comforting, healing or therapeutic. We all have experienced a hand that caresses us, and in this experience we know how the caress brings about a change in the hand. A caress transforms the body, suggests Buytendijk (1970), even if the physiologist is unable to report on this transformation. Sometimes we may feel that our body is more or less foreign to us: why do I have this particular body? these eyes? this nose? these hands? But then when another person touches us—in friendship, care or love—the contingencies of our own body are eliminated. A justification of the body takes place. The touch removes the distance between two bodies and one is invited to be one with one's own body, to inhabit one's own body.

Precisely because this private, sometimes intimate touch can accomplish so much, there exists an uncomfortable ambiguity. The intimate touch is what the student nurses in Jean van der Zalm's story referred to as 'unprofessional'; it was the touch they feared because it might have been misinterpreted by the patient. Also, practising palpation on each other left open all kinds of possibilities for ambiguity for the student nurses. How can I submit my self-conscious body to the scrutinising palpation of my classmate without feeling touched in an intimate manner? Similarly, in palpating the body of my fellow student, how can I pretend that this is just a body, a body without a person, a person who feels somewhat embarrassed and exposed under a hospital gown?

The same is true in real nursing situations—a light palpation of the skin might be experienced by the patient as caressing, as too intimate. So, it seems that the private touch may render the nurse–patient relationship ambiguous. The private touch might mean that the hand that touches has a special interest in the other. Again, this may manifest itself in significations of embarrassment.

The personal pathic touch

The personal pathic touch, which the medical texts on palpation do not mention, is evident in Jean's story through the patient's positive response to the nurse's comforting hand. Of course, the private touch is also pathic, but the special quality of the nurse's hand meant that her touch was not private but 'professional' in intent. The pathic hand, and the pathic knowledge that supports it, could be seen to lie at the heart of nursing practice, since its effect is to reunite or reintegrate the patient with his or her body. Thus the gnostic aspect of health science works in the opposite direction to the pathic. The gnostically healing attitude analyses, anatomises, dissects and makes diagnoses and prognoses that tend to separate us from our body, so to speak. The pathically healing attitude of nursing aims to console and comfort, to wake in times of suffering, to be there in moments of need, to support in the process of convalescence. And so it aims to assist the recovering patient in feeling whole and make life liveable again, even if sometimes under the constraints of chronic difficulties.

The word 'pathic' derives from 'pathos', meaning 'suffering', and also passion and disease or 'a quality that arouses pity or sorrow'. In a larger life context, the pathic refers to the general mood, sensibility and felt sense of being in the world. As in the example with breathing, Buytendijk (1974) draws a close relation between the pathic experience and the mood of the lived body. The pathically tuned body perceives the world in a feeling or emotive way.

Strangely perhaps, the very notion of touch presupposes our lived distance from things and others. Without touch it would not be possible to go away, to let go, or to lose contact and to get in touch again (Buytendijk 1970, p. 100). This also means that touch is the primordial medium by which to overcome separation and relational distance. Neither the ear nor the eye can give us an experience of human contact in the same pathically direct manner as touch. Indeed we may be deeply moved by a human voice or a meaningful glance, but the touch stirs us in a particularly intimate manner. It may even happen at times that we are touched to tears—as in the case of the elderly patient and nurse above.

Heidegger uses the notion of *Befindlichkeit* to refer to this sense that we have of ourselves in certain situations. Literally, *Befindlichkeit* means 'the way one finds oneself' in the world. We have an implicit, felt understanding of ourselves in situations even though it is difficult sometimes to put that understanding into words. The therapist Gendlin (1988, p. 45) suggests that this kind of understanding is not cognitive in the usual sense: 'It is sensed or felt, rather than thought—and it may not even be sensed or felt directly with attention.' And yet, our sense of the pathic in our own or in other people's existence can become a topic for our phenomenological reflection. The important point for phenomenological inquiry is that cognitive insights by themselves cannot address non-cognitive meaning. Thus we may need to employ non-cognitive as well as cognitive methods in order to address pathic experience.

ON THE RELEVANCE OF PATHIC INQUIRY FOR NURSING PRACTICE

So wherein lie some of the differences between gnostic and pathic thought and practice? When we compare the more gnostic medical relation to the more pathic nursing relation, we note that medical diagnostic practice first of all searches for symptomatic clues and determining factors in the patient's history. For example, the medical specialist may look for causal, symptomatic or developmental patterns, for a difficult birth, for psychological, physical and genetic abnormalities in parents, grandparents and other close family members. Psychiatric clinical thought operates in a similar manner: one undertakes psychological analyses, administers diagnostic instruments and applies intelligence tests, personality inventories and other measuring devices. One searches for disease patterns *by looking back* into personal and family histories.

Thus, the gnostic mode of thinking and practising leads to a certain idea of the meaning of healing: the gnostic approach is to locate the pathology and then to 'cut out' the intrusion that has been festering there for days, weeks or even years. Just as one frees someone from his or her appendix in the medical room, so one searches for and removes the 'psychological problem' by 'cutting it out' of people's lives in the therapeutic room. How is this experienced by the patient? Sometimes it may seem that in the process of diagnosis, the physician, the psychologist, the psychiatrist 'gives' the patient a tumour, a neurosis, a paranoia. And, of course, once the patient has been given the illness, then medical treatment consists of cutting it out again.

A feature of the medicalisation of increasing aspects of life and body functions is that the gnostic act tends to fragment. When a disease has been treated properly, when a surgical operation has been completed successfully, this does not mean necessarily that the patient has been reintegrated with his or her body or with his or her world. This is exactly where pathic practice enters. In this way the pathic nursing act complements the gnostic medical act, in the sense that the pathic meaning of nursing consists of reuniting the patient with his or her body, thus making life liveable again in whatever way this has to be learned by the patient. For example, in the everydayness of nursing the pathic processes of taking patients to the bathroom, prompting them to get out of bed and encouraging personal hygiene are performed in the awareness that they have to do with relationships and with the re-establishing of relationships. One nurse said: 'When

I see the patient look in the mirror then I know that the healing is in progress, that the patient is getting better.'[4]

Of course, it would be wrong to suggest that the gnostic approach of the medical doctor would preclude a meaningful caring relation. 'The "gnostic" contact should not be interpreted as a cold, calculating, dry and therefore heartless association with the patient,' says Van den Berg (1980, p. 131). But it may be true, as Van den Berg proposes, that the sense of caring and trust is different for the medical doctor, who sees the patient only briefly, and for the nurse, who hopefully is present or available throughout a period of time. The patient tends to experience the physician with a different 'nearness', a nearness which is due not to pathic qualities but to the 'knowing relationship of the doctor and his patient . . . The medical contact combines a maximum of trust with a minimum of familiarity.' (Van den Berg 1980, p. 131) Is Van den Berg suggesting that the gnostic contact may nevertheless be experienced differently from the caring attentiveness of the nurse? In the text *The Psychology of the Sickbed* (Van den Berg 1980), the nurse is strangely absent from his account. And yet, it is in the different kind of trust between the pathic and the gnostic quality of the contact as well as in the 'hand' that the difference between the medical and the nursing relation may be sought.

I need to trust with confidence the knowing, palpating hand that skilfully probes my skin for what is underneath. In our culture and age the specialist physician's hand is primarily the *gnostic* hand, a knowing intellectual hand, a hand of science, as it (dia)gnostically examines the body for signs of trouble, or as it surgically operates on the body to remove a feared tumour. The physician's hand makes me aware that I am made up of internal organs and that I can take distance from my body as if it were a mere vessel for my soul.

If I have confidence in the physician then I experience the palpating medical hand as an instrument of competence in whose knowledge and skills and healing powers I trust. But this confidential trust is quite one-sided; there are other kinds of trust that depend on the strength of mutual, two-sided human relationships. Bollnow (1989) has clarified the phenomenological difference between *confidence* and pure *trust*. Confidence is less dependent on relationality and the intrinsic moral character of trust, says Bollnow. Confidence is basically concerned with performance, specific competencies and expert skills. For example, from the patient's point of view it is reassuring to have confidence in one's surgeon, but from the surgeon's point of view, his or her expertise is not really dependent upon the patient's confidence.

In contrast with the knowing or gnostic hand of palpation, the nurse's hand is pathic when it applies the dressing, straightens the bedding, starts an intravenous infusion, administers medication, cleans the skin, provides relief from pain, supports the aching body in its time of healing. True, the nurse's hand is also knowledgeable of medical science. But (outside of highly technologised intensive care, emergency or technical tasks) the patient still expects that the nurse's hand is primarily a healing hand, a caring hand which touches not only the physical body, but also the self, the whole embodied person. This pathic quality may well constitute the core meaning of the healing act of nursing care. If, as a patient, I trust this hand, then it has the power to reunite me pathically with my body, reminding me that I am one with my body and thus making it possible for me to heal, to strengthen, to become whole.

This contrasts with the cognitive confidence that we must have in the medical expert or surgeon. The medical hand may rid my body of a malignant intruder, provide lifesaving assistance or perform a complicated technical task. And yet, these procedures may leave my life profoundly disturbed.

How is the nurse's hand expressive, potentially at least, of the caring, pathic relation? The pathic relation demands a very personal involvement. At the same time, the nurse's hand, especially in bedside practice, always has at least a double function: simultaneously gnostic and pathic, instrumental and caring. It seems that it is difficult to capture the ambiguity of the nursing hand and the nursing relation. In our languages the pathic is ultimately unnameable and easily slips away.

Of course, this gnostic–pathic ambiguity can arise in many healthcare situations. For example, a physiotherapist may manipulate or massage a patient's body with gnostic intent while the patient would say that the treatment has the quality of a pathic experience. Many medical procedures that are primarily technical may give the patient a pathic trust in the physician, especially if the quality of the relationship between the patient and doctor is personal.

What then makes pathic practice distinct? The difference is this: pathic thought turns itself immediately and directly to the person. A pathic relation is always specific and unique. Even a relatively brief encounter between a patient and a healthcare provider can have this personal quality. A personal relation is something we can have only with a specific other. The pathic orientation meets this concrete person in the heart of his or her existence, without trying to reduce the person to a diagnostic picture, a certain kind of case, a preconceived category of patient, a psychological type, a set of factors on a scale or a theoretical classification. In other words, there is something deeply personal or intersubjective to the pathic relation. This is the reason why the pathic personal relation is easily confused with the private one.

What is pathically quite compelling is the way in which any particular person fails to match preconceived gnostic distinctions, diagnostic judgements and prognostic projections. How with any particular patient the clinical path of an illness is always different from medical assessment. How the experience of disease is never experienced in exactly the same manner by different persons. How patients often continue to live when they were supposed to die or die when they were expected to recover.

This constant 'defying difference' between diagnosis or prognosis on the one hand and contingency and concreteness on the other, is what makes each person, each patient, uniquely who he or she is—which is never the same as the diagnostic portrait that the expert constructs. The individual human being always falls to a certain extent 'outside' of the dossier, the diagnosis, the description, the prognosis.[5]

If we want to be sensitive to the pathic nature of nursing and medical practice then we need to pursue forms of research that use pathic language. Pathic questions cannot be answered by texts that primarily communicate cognitive meaning. And gnostic insights cannot produce pathic experience. To construct texts that can address and reflect on the experience of illness we need to get beyond the objectifying effects of naming the things of our world with labels that distance us from them. We need to write (and read) for tone and pathic understanding and, to this effect, our words must be slow, new, single and tentative.

NOTES

1. The English word 'surname' is a bit misleading since it is really the first name that is added to the family name.
2. I thank Jean van der Zalm for sharing her experiences and course materials with me.
3. I thank Dr Tom Magson and Teresa Dobson for this account.
4. I thank Yvonne Hayne and Jean van der Zalm for some helpful discussions.
5. See especially Beets (1952) for an explication of these distinctions in the realm of psychology.

REFERENCES

Beets, N. 1952 *Verstandhouding en Onderscheid* Boom Meppel, Amsterdam

Bollnow, O.F. 1989 'The pedagogical atmosphere: the perspective of the educator' *Phenomenology + Pedagogy* vol. 7, pp. 37–63

Buytendijk, F.J.J. 1970 'Some aspects of touch' *Journal of Phenomenological Psychology* vol. 1, no. 1, pp. 99–124

——1974 *Prolegomena to an Anthropological Physiology* Duquesne University Press, Pittsburgh, Pa.

Clarke, M. 1997 'Memories of breathing: asthma as a way of becoming' *Textorium* Human Science Project Publication, Edmonton, Canada

DeGowin, E.L. & DeGowin, R.L. 1976 *Bedside Diagnostic Examination* Macmillan, New York

Derrida, J. 1995 *On the Name* Stanford University Press, Stanford, Ca.

Gendlin, E.T. 1988 'Befindlichkeit: Heidegger and the philosophy of psychology' in *Review of Existential Psychology and Psychiatry* (special issue, *Heidegger and Psychology* ed. K. Heller)

Heidegger, M. 1962 *Being and Time* Harper & Row, New York

——1971 *Poetry, Language, Thought* Harper & Row, New York

Kot, P. (n.d.) *An Overview of Physical Examination Techniques* course handout, Nursing 104, Faculty of Nursing, University of Alberta, Canada

Le Guin, U.K. 1987 'She unnames them' *Buffalo Gals and Other Animal Presences* Penguin, Markham, Ontario, pp. 194–6

Merleau-Ponty, M. 1962 *Phenomenology of Perception* Routledge & Kegan Paul, London

——1964 *Signs* Northwestern University Press, Evanston, Ill.

Van den Berg, J.H. 1959 *Het Menselijk Lichaam* Callenbach, Nijkerk

——1972 *A Different Existence* Duquesne University Press, Pittsburgh, Pa. (Originally published in 1964 as *De Psychiatrische Patient* Callenbach, Nijkerk)

——1980 *The Psychology of the Sickbed* Humanities Press, New York

——1987 'The meaning of being ill' in *Phenomenological Psychology: The Dutch School* ed. J.J. Kockelmans, Martinus Nijhoff Publishers, Dordrecht/Boston, pp. 229–38

three

On living with chronic leg ulcers

MARIAN BLAND

The Heideggarian phenomenological study on which this chapter is based was undertaken to complete the requirements of a Masters in Nursing in New Zealand. The study question was: 'What is it like to live with chronic leg ulcers?'

The five male and four female participants in the study ranged in age from 56 to 81 years. They were all clients of a community nursing service in a large provincial city in New Zealand, who were undergoing treatment for leg ulcers that had been present for between six months to over six years.

No attempt was made to establish the aetiology of the ulcers, as the emphasis of the study was on experiences, rather than on leg ulcer management. Cullum's (1994, p. 3) definition of leg ulcers as 'tissue breakdown on the leg or foot due to any cause' was adopted for the purposes of the study.

Six of the participants had experienced leg ulcers previously, including two who had shared their lives with leg ulcers for more than 43 years and 47 years respectively. Multiple semi-structured interviews were used to reveal the experiences of the participants with both their current and previous ulcers.

The existential lifeworld themes of lived body, lived other, temporality and spatiality (van Manen 1990) were used as the framework around which to structure the results of the hermeneutic interpretation of the participants' stories. All names used are fictional, though in a few instances, where comments are thought to leave the person particularly vulnerable to identification, names have been withheld.

I FIRST BECAME aware that leg ulcers were a significant problem when I began working as a district nurse nine years ago. Within a very short time I realised just how much of my day was spent dressing leg ulcers, and how difficult it was to heal these wounds permanently, if at all. My interest in leg ulcers initially originated from a desire to increase the effectiveness of my wound management practices, partly because of the sympathy I felt for these patients, but also to reduce the demands they made on nursing time and resources.

I was conscious that I knew little of recent developments in wound management, and when the opportunity arose during my university studies to undertake a literature review on a topic of my choice, leg ulcer management was an obvious selection.

Around the same time, again as part of my university studies, I was introduced to the phenomenological work of Benner and Wrubel (1989). I became increasingly aware of how important it is that nurses understand patients' experiences of illness, and how little was currently known of these experiences.

When I began the literature review I originally regretted my choice of topic, for there is a vast amount of literature relating to leg ulcers. Gradually I came to realise that despite all this literature, these mountains of words, virtually nothing existed on the patient's perspective of the experience, on what it was like to live with these ulcers. Everything I read about leg ulcers was related to what health professionals saw as the problems, such as the prevalence of ulcers, the difficulties of wound management, the costs associated with their treatment, and alleged non-compliance with treatment regimes. Until recently, little attempt had been made to understand the illness experiences associated with this condition, an understanding that would facilitate the provision of patient-focused not wound-focused care. I began talking to patients with leg ulcers and soon realised that, although I might have been visiting them on a frequent (even daily) basis for many months, I actually knew little of how their ulcers had impacted on their lives and how they had coped over the years.

SIGNIFICANCE OF THE STUDY

There are no published studies of the prevalence of leg ulcers in New Zealand, although overseas studies indicate open ulcers in 0.15 per cent of the general population, with a history of ulceration in approximately 4 per cent of the population over 65 (Callam et al. 1988). While the total number of people with leg ulcers may be relatively small, it is the chronic nature of the condition that makes these ulcers so significant for the individual concerned, and also for the health professionals involved in their management. The lengthy duration of the ulcers and the repeated episodes of ulceration are demonstrated by Baker et al. (1991). Of the 138 participants in their study, 76 per cent had experienced previous ulceration; of these 28 per cent had experienced more than ten episodes of ulceration, while 46 per cent of the current ulcers had been present for longer than 26 weeks. Over 50 per cent of the 382 participants in the study by Nelzen et al. (1994) had current ulcers of more than one year's duration, with 20 per cent of those ulcers being larger than 10 cm in size.

The chronic nature of the wounds and the difficulties inherent in achieving a permanent cure have obviously been the source of considerable frustration for some health professionals. That frustration has at times been evident in attitudes to and opinions expressed about people with leg ulcers. As several authors (Ertl 1992; Hamer et al. 1994; Lindholm et al. 1993) discuss, there is an oft-quoted belief that many patients do not want their ulcers to heal because they will lose contact with the district nurses, and hence they may in fact deliberately prolong treatment. The comment by Wise (1986, p. 39) is typical: 'Her ulcer has healed twice in the past two years but recurred within two months of healing . . . so it is probably a factitious ulcer which she uses to ensure regular contact.' Cullum (1994, p. 62) also discusses the notion that leg ulcer patients do not want their ulcers to heal, but comments that '*there has been no evidence published to substantiate these impressions*'.

The financial costs associated with chronic leg ulcers is becoming a motivating force for healthcare providers to establish more effective treatment regimes. There is limited acknowledgement of the problems associated with the ulcers—such as wound odour, pain and loss of mobility—as the human costs associated with living with chronic leg ulcers have been largely ignored by researchers (Charles 1995; Hamer et al. 1994).

LIVING WITH A BODY THAT CAN NO LONGER BE RELIED UPON

Chronic leg ulcers are evidence of a breakdown in the normal 'smooth functioning of the body' (Benner & Wrubel 1989, p. 59). This breakdown impacts on the body in two ways—the body is out of control, and treatment regimens alter the person's sense of embodiment by restricting previously taken-for-granted habits and routines and altering bodily sensations.

An inability to control the body is demonstrated by the pain, odour and ooze that characterise chronic leg ulcers. For, despite the best efforts of participants to adhere strictly to the prescribed treatments, these wounds appear to continue almost at will—wounds fail to heal, new ulcers begin and wound infections recur with disappointing regularity.

Pain is a universal feature of the leg ulcer experience, although the nature and intensity of the pain varies greatly. The level of pain experienced may range from general discomfort to pain so severe that even walking becomes impossible. Don said:

> *I was laid up for four months—I couldn't even get off the couch. I had to crawl to the toilet—I had a really bad one [ulcer].*

Jim became '*so sick and tired of the pain*' that he requested the amputation of his leg. Similarly, pain was a significant factor in Gary's decision to finally proceed with amputation:

> *Those pills got immune in the end—pain started creeping through . . . I came in and said to them, 'I can't stand the pain any longer—take it off.'*

The pain associated with venous ulcers can be more intermittent, but still cause considerable discomfort:

> *But [sighs] just now and again they grip—the pain grips and throbs where the ulcers are, just now and again. The left leg goes, and then it tells the right leg to go.* (Hugh)

In addition to the pain that arises directly from the condition itself, pain may also be clinically inflicted during dressing changes—as the old dressings are removed, when wounds are cleaned roughly, if the wound is exposed to the air for any period of time, as the new dressing is applied.

I'm always glad when it is finished. Because you see they put that thick thing on [hydrocolloid dressing], and then they sort of press it down with their hands—it hurts when they put pressure on it, but they have to do that to make the stuff stick on the skin. (Hugh)

Study participants often had difficulty in articulating the pain they experienced. The nature, frequency and intensity of the pain varied considerably for individuals over time, and participants were reluctant to dwell on this topic. Pain becomes something to get used to, something to learn to live with.

Something else to get used to are wound infections, which are common despite strict attention to aseptic dressing techniques on the part of the nurses and the care taken by the participants to maintain home hygiene. Wound infections usually mean an increase in pain and a delay in wound healing. One of the greatest drawbacks with a wound infection is the need for antibiotic therapy. One study participant had been prescribed eighteen different courses of antibiotics over a two-year period. Side effects from antibiotics, such as nausea and vomiting, are not infrequent:

And I started taking those [antibiotics] and I felt terribly sick—I felt the veins right across my stomach, and sick . . . But I felt that miserable, I didn't care what they did—I felt I wanted to die. Anyway, after that happened they gave me a white tablet, a little white tablet [anti-emetic], and I had to take that a half an hour before I took the antibiotic capsule, and then an hour after I took that I could have my meals. It was a bit of a nark [nuisance], because I had to have the alarm clock for half-past seven to take my tablet so I could have my breakfast by nine. (Hugh)

Despite the side effects experienced with antibiotics, wound infections are ignored at one's own peril, as the potential for serious infection, and subsequent amputation, is always present.

Wounds oozing out onto bandages, clothing and even bed linen was another problem that had been experienced by all study participants at some time:

It looks so dirty, filthy when they [bandages] are looking all brown, and they get darker and darker. Well, it's not nice to look at really . . . I mean, it's not just a little mark, sometimes it's right round my leg. (Connie)

Leaking wounds not only look unsightly, but also mean having to deal with the laundering of filthy, soiled bandages and sometimes sheets. For those no longer able to do their own laundry, this may mean the shame of letting others deal with the mess. Extensive precautions are taken to protect the surrounding environment from being soiled. Often, wounds are re-dressed just before retiring at night or extra padding is applied. Despite this, leaking of wounds out onto bed linen is still a great concern.

Going away from home when wounds are leaking copiously is at the very least fraught with tension, and at worst impossible. Used dressings must be disposed of and soiled bandages laundered, and there is an ever-present fear that wounds will leak out onto somebody else's sheets.

Having a body that smells is difficult to ignore. Particularly at times of wound infections or copious wound exudate, the fear of offending others is very real and compounds the unpleasantness for participants of being able to smell their own wounds:

> *Oh, I think, yeah, the worst part would be just occasionally when you get the smell, and you can't get home and you can't change, and . . . [voice trails off]. I suppose people think you have got b.o. [body odour] or something. You know, if it's starting to smell you have got that when you go to bed at night too, and then my wife has to put up with it too.* (Jim)

For Gary, the months prior to the amputation of his leg were filled with a constant awareness of the wound odour, and the impact it had on others. Gary described the wound odour as 'a putrid, sickly smell, a smell you could taste in your mouth'. He became so self-conscious about the smell that he would wait outside in the hospital corridor at clinic appointments rather than risk offending others in the waiting room.

Wound odour is minimised when occlusive dressing products are used, because the exudate is contained. However, when those dressings are being changed there is a sudden awareness of the smell of the wound. And there is always the worry that if wounds leak out before the next scheduled dressing change other people will also be able to smell them.

Having chronic wounds means being trapped in a body that is imperfect. A part of the body has broken down and stubbornly refuses to be repaired. In fact, the body may behave badly and be a source of social embarrassment by smelling and leaking out in a relatively uncontrollable manner. The uncertainty of how the body will behave makes social interaction difficult and restricts the ability to plan ahead because of the unpredictability of what the body will be doing at that time.

Some aspects of the disease process itself are particularly unpleasant and difficult to adjust to, like the pain and the vulnerability to wound infections associated with the disease process. Alterations to embodiment are also experienced when treatments disrupt one's being-in-the-world. Having a shower may now require almost military-style planning to protect the wound, unsightly and uncomfortable bandages restrict footwear options, and the advice to rest the limb poses almost insurmountable problems in relation to carrying out the activities of daily living and maintaining a sense of wellbeing.

THE IMPACT OF TREATMENT REGIMENS

Having a bath or shower when leg ulcers are present can become a major event. There are now a number of waterproof dressing products available, but the majority of the study participants wore dressings that needed to be kept dry, so that having a bath or shower required care and planning. Archie had a waterproof dressing on his wound, but he was still limited to showering only on the two days a week on which the district nurses visited because he could not reapply the bandage himself. A daily shower or bath had been his lifetime practice, and the restriction of this activity to twice a week was keenly felt.

Edna had her shower with her leg encased in a plastic bag, and washed her foot separately later:

> *But I'd love to be able to put it [her foot] under the shower and say, 'here shower, wash it'. It feels as though, no matter how many times I've sponged it, it never feels clean. Because I get very embarrassed about foot odours.*

Only one participant mentioned the district nurses washing the leg when changing the dressings. For most, it was never a routine part of the dressing changes and, as some nurses would never offer to wash the leg, weeks could go by without it being done.

The combination of summer heat and toe-to-knee bandages or compression stockings is not always a happy one, particularly when the opportunity for showering is limited. This physical discomfort that accompanies the bandages makes compliance a problem:

> *Having the bandage on, on hot days, that's not comfortable. I think one has to keep it on to assist the healing process, but then again, some days I take it off—it becomes unbearable. You feel as though you want to be like a kid with a broken arm—get something and rub it up underneath the bandage.* (Archie)

Study participants appeared to have a good understanding of the importance of bandages in wound management. Appreciating why bandages were necessary meant Edna was particularly conscientious about following advice from her general practitioner (family physician):

> *I'm all right when I'm lying on the bed, but as soon as I go to get up I have to put the bandage on. Because they said, every time I go to walk, that's when you do the damage. So when I get up in the middle of the night to go to the toilet I have to put the bandage on, and when I go to get back into bed off comes the bandage again and I have to sit there and roll it all up into a roll so it's easy to put on the first thing in the morning.*

Having layers of bandages around the foot and lower leg may mean shoes no longer fit or get stretched out of shape, while the unsightly bandages may be considered likely to attract unwanted attention. Compression stockings are now replacing bandages for venous leg ulcers, resulting in fewer difficulties with footwear. But applying and taking off these stockings can be very difficult to manage independently.

Bandaging and resting the limb were the two mainstays of ulcer treatment for study participants. All had been advised to rest, but sometimes little information was given on how this was to be achieved or what period of time should be aimed for. The advice to 'rest' posed many difficulties. Life must go on, and household responsibilities continue:

> *It's all right for some people, because they might have someone live in the house who can do for them, and they can rest their legs. They can have their meals cooked for them and everything. But I have to do it myself, my own washing and everything.* (Hugh)

As Jim was the main breadwinner for the family, the need for him to continue in paid employment meant that rest was almost impossible:

> *When I first got it [the ulcer] they said that's the only way you are going to heal it—get your feet off the floor. But I was a manual worker and I couldn't do much about that [sighs deeply].*

When a choice is necessary between living for today or making changes that will pay off at some future time, it can be difficult to decide which should be paramount. Even when priorities are adjusted so that resting is possible, the enforced inactivity may provide an unwelcome opportunity to reflect on the things that need doing.

Accepting advice to keep the leg elevated when leg ulcers are a chronic condition could mean a drastic alteration to lifestyle. Most study participants appear to have reached a compromise: normal activities are undertaken as much as the pain will allow; at the same time a conscious effort is made to fit in a specific rest period sometime during the day.

THE BODY IN TIME AND SPACE

Benner and Wrubel (1989, p. 64) contrast the Western notion of time as 'a linear succession of moments' with the existential concept of temporality, which they define as 'the way the person simultaneously lives in the present, is influenced by the past, and is projected in the future' (1989, pp. 412–13). The experience of ulcers in the past helps shape the way current ulcers are experienced, and offers both hope and fear for the future.

The chronic nature of the leg ulcer experience can mean that even in the absence of current ulcers, the potential for their development in the future is such that ulcers are effectively always present. At the same time, interpretations of chronological age are distorted by the physical impact of the ulcers—a consciousness develops of the ageing process such that patients perceive themselves as aged and see this as a factor in delayed healing.

Two of the study participants have lived with leg ulcers for the majority of the past four decades, and another three participants have had their lives disrupted by leg ulcers for more than five years. Although chronic in duration, the wounds themselves are dynamic in nature, with constant cycles of deterioration, of new ulcers forming and of wounds healing. Improvements may be slow and difficult to discern but regular measuring of wounds by nurses gives some indication of progress. The deterioration of wounds, meanwhile, is usually much more dramatic, sometimes seeming to occur virtually overnight.

As the body can no longer be trusted to behave, there is a certain suspense when dressings are changed, particularly when new treatments are being used. What will be revealed this time? Edna told of her disappointment after her nurse had tried a new dressing product overnight:

> *Well, it had dried up good. Well, the next day she came, and it had all broken out again, all flamed up, sore and red.*

Setbacks and disappointments are commonplace. In particular, skin grafting raises hopes of a reasonably quick end to the ulcers—hopes that can be dashed when grafts fail to take. Hugh spent six weeks in hospital, and during this period his ulcers were grafted twice. He was interviewed two days after returning home and was asked how confident he felt that those second grafts would be successful:

> *These ulcers are up and down [sighs heavily]. I mean, they look as if they are coming right and then they take a turn for the worse. As I say, when I came home the girl [district nurse] just touched it and it oozed, and it hadn't oozed for days. But I think by this time they should have taken. That worries me a little bit.*

For elderly study participants, leg ulcers had the effect of emphasising physical deterioration, described by Archie as 'old age creeping up on me, from the legs up'. Physical fitness is harder to maintain as one ages, a situation that is not helped by the advice to rest for lengthy periods. When physical frailty means a daily battle to retain independence and continue living at home, there is a wariness of doing anything that might jeopardise that independence.

For those who have had leg ulcers before, unpleasant experiences can be recalled and used to interpret current situations, such as the suspicion or dread that the current delay in wound healing may indicate the presence of an infection:

> *Because [you] don't want an infection in them [donor sites on thighs] again, you can't bear to have them bathed, you can't bear to have dressings on. It's dreadful, really dreadful, very painful.* (Connie)

Past events and lifestyles are re-examined in order to try to find some explanation for the development of the ulcers. In general, the study participants felt that the ulcers were due to factors beyond their control, such as diabetes or accidental injury. Sometimes no explanation was obvious:

> *I have asked the Lord upstairs, 'What have I done to deserve this?' . . . It surprises me, where do I get it from?* (Freda)

With first ulcers, the inability to predict what will happen means little or no progress is particularly difficult to deal with:

> *Well the doctor said he had a woman in with exactly the same thing that I had, and yet hers was cleared up in a month. Why was mine still going six months later? What did she do that I haven't done to get hers cleared up so quick? [Laughs bitterly.] I wish I had been given*

her phone number so I could ring her and ask her what she did to get hers cleared up. (Edna)

Although over time a degree of acceptance about the ulcers may develop, this does not mean that hope of permanent wound healing is abandoned, and all participants remained open to trying new dressing products, hopeful of a 'miracle cure' just around the corner.

Some participants were realistic enough to acknowledge that their ulcers may never heal, and may deteriorate to the extent that amputation of the limb would be required. The possibility of amputation is obviously a very distressing prospect, and ethical concerns limited how deeply this topic could be pursued during the study. Amputation was only discussed with participants when it was evident from their comments that they had already considered this eventuality for themselves. Avoidance of the word 'amputation' was obvious, with the term 'gangrene' being used by many participants instead, which suggests that the issue is almost too awful to contemplate. The possibility of amputation was not obvious to Gary, and he failed to heed medical advice about changing his lifestyle:

Yeah I was warned, but as I said, I've got painted-on ears. I've come to understand that if I had listened in the first place and did all I was supposed to do I wouldn't have had it [amputation].

When an ulcer does finally heal, the possibility of further ulcers developing means that vigilance is always required. Care must still be taken to protect the limbs, and the legs are constantly monitored for any signs that a new ulcer may be forming. The ulcers never go away and victory over the wounds is only temporary, with the next ulcer waiting just around the corner. A future without ulcers is difficult to imagine.

INCREASING THE NEED FOR PERSONAL SPACE

When there has been a history of leg ulcers the possibility of certain procedures and treatments needing to be repeated can cause concern and even dread. Study participants were aware of just how easy it was to accidentally aggravate an existing wound or start a new ulcer, and hence of the need to protect the body by increasing personal space. Routines were altered and some social activities abandoned in order to avoid situations of potential danger. Venturing outside the home means exposure to potential injury. Busy shopping days must be avoided because of the challenge posed by wayward supermarket trolleys. Activities previously enjoyed may have to be abandoned because personal safety cannot be guaranteed. Wounds can be very painful if knocked, and much energy is expended in trying to protect them.

During the day the body can be monitored and precautions can be taken, but this control is more difficult at night. The pressure of bedclothes is frequently a problem, and a variety of solutions were used by study participants to overcome this, like placing rolled-up towels at the foot of the bed, or constructing bed cradles out of cardboard boxes. Connie had a more novel solution:

> *I've had all sorts of things to try to keep the blankets off. At the moment I've got a packet of eight toilet rolls. It doesn't fall over because of the double layer—it keeps it in place.*

After years of taking care that his legs did not get knocked, Don and his wife found it easier to resort to single beds. The need for increased personal space around the body requires constant vigilance of both the self and others. For even in the relative safety of home, the body is still not safe. Particular care must still be taken to position the body in such a way as to avoid pressure on the wound, especially at night.

When outings are curtailed by the need to rest the leg or because of the pain experienced when mobilising, the potential exists for the home to become a kind of prison—with a sofa becoming the centre of a very restricted universe. Health professionals are usually welcomed, but their visits also open the home (and its inhabitants) to scrutiny and potential judgement.

THE IMPACT OF THE BODY ON RELATIONSHIPS WITH OTHERS

When there are problems with the body breaking down, such as with the development of leg ulcers, new relationships are formed and existing relationships change. The assistance of health professionals is required to help treat the wounds. The relationships formed with health professionals are complex—to some extent they necessitate the 'handing over' of control to those who are perceived as (or hoped to be) experts. Care must be taken not to offend these experts, and lifestyles are altered as far as possible to accommodate the rules the experts set.

The long-term management of leg ulcers in New Zealand is largely the domain of the district nursing service, with nurses visiting on a regular, sometimes daily basis, for what may be lengthy periods of time. Nurses were described by study participants as 'struggling for years' to heal the ulcers, and were seen to be working to achieve the best possible wound management.

Wound healing was perceived by participants to be largely out of their control. It is the treatments applied by health professionals to the wound which generates results. It was not uncommon to hear specific nurses being credited with healing a particular wound. It was therefore very important to participants that 'their nurse' had the expertise to heal wounds, a confidence reinforced when other health professionals also acknowledged that expertise:

> *She [district nurse] is the only one I've been able to understand and she seems to know what she is talking about, and when I mentioned to the doctor that I had her, he said, 'Oh, she's good.'* (Edna)

Frequent contact over a lengthy period sometimes results in strong friendships being established, particularly when the nurses extend their concern to other family members, acknowledging the impact the ulcers have had on them as well. However, while developing a close personal relationship with a particular nurse is valued, there can be problems when it is necessary for the client to be 'handed over' to another district nursing team. As well as coping with the loss of that personal relationship, the new nurse(s) may not be perceived as having similar competence:

> *One of them [new nurses] came yesterday for the first time and she dressed it all the way round—where you are not supposed to—and taped it all the way round. [The previous nurse] was good. She just sort of daubs it, washes it, daubs it lightly—but the one yesterday, she was scratch, scratch, scrape like that, and it was quite sore when she had finished.* (Name withheld)

It was not unusual for nurses to have different ideas about how the wounds should be managed:

> *Well, the nurses are all very good, but they all have their own ideas of what they should use. There is [sic] no two nurses that are the same. Even to the way they put bandages on.* (Connie)

While participants were generally very positive about the services provided by the district nurses, not all their interactions were helpful. Two study participants saw personality clashes as being almost inevitable. Comments were also made by some about their lack of choice over which district nurse they had, with one person talking about 'dreading one or two particular nurses turning up'.

Van Manen (1990, p. 102) describes home as the place 'where we can *be* what *we are*'. While the input of the district nurses may be welcomed, their regular visits still invade the privacy of the home.

> *They come so often they get to know the house, they just roam around as if . . . They are quite at home—I just let them go.* (Connie)

By opening their homes to visiting nurses, people can feel as if their homes, and everyone in them, are being laid open to the scrutiny and potential judgement of others:

> *'She [district nurse] asked to use the toilet here one day, and we thought oh yes—we had the same thought about it—she must have thought we were clean people.* (Don)

Family doctors, the nurses associated with their practices and hospital specialists can also be involved in wound management. There were differing opinions among the study participants about the knowledge and expertise of family doctors, who appeared to have little involvement in the day-to-day management of the wounds. Only Edna saw her doctor on a regular (fortnightly) basis, and seeing him so frequently was not always helpful:

> *And he says, 'Oh, I don't know what we are going to put on that,' and 'I don't know what we are going to do with this.' And then she [practice nurse] is reading a chart on the wall to see what dressing to put on.* (Edna)

The authority of specialists was respected by all the participants. Even though specialists may prescribe unpopular remedies (such as skin grafting), in the end it was felt that there was no option but to comply as far as possible with instructions:

> *You do go along with it in the hope that he's got enough brains to know what he is doing. He should know what he is doing, and therefore you trust him.* (Betty)

But there is an unequal balance of power between the parties. Accepting the professionals as experts means there is an obligation to try to comply with the recommended treatments even though individuals may have accumulated considerable knowledge and expertise about their wounds over the years. When health professionals are involved, individuals may effectively surrender control of the wound:

> *[The bandages] slip and slide and of course I'm not allowed to take them off or do anything . . . I'm not allowed to take the underneath one off.*
>
> (Can you change your own dressings if you need to?)
>
> *They won't let me do that. They used to at one time, but not now.* (Name withheld)

Surrendering control means having to accept, or work within, the rules set by the health professionals. Sometimes a certain tension exists, when rules are acknowledged but the body-aware-of-itself is making other demands:

> *Nobody knows my body like I do. If my body wants a good wash, a good shower it gets it. I'll do everything in my power so that I can do that. No other person can tell me what I should do, because I feel like it, I want it, I'll have it.* (Archie)

A balancing act is required—acknowledging the requirements dictated by the body, but taking care not to antagonise health professionals.

There is the potential for conflict to arise over wound management when there are various health professionals involved. The client is in the middle, struggling with divided loyalties and wondering whose advice to follow:

> *[The nurse] this morning told me I'm better if I get up and do a bit of exercise, and yet the doctor told me to lie down all day with my legs elevated higher than my heart. And yet here is one this morning telling me I'm better if I get up and do a bit of walking.*
>
> (So how does that make you feel?)
>
> *As though I don't know which way to turn! I'm trying to please everybody and I don't seem to be getting anywhere.* (Edna)

CONTINUING ON WITH LIFE

Reflecting on the experiences outlined thus far, it would be easy to regard the chronic leg ulcer experience as involving never-ending misery and distress. This would not be an accurate portrayal of the lives of all but one of the study participants. Life has continued on for them, despite the interruptions the ulcers have caused. The ulcers have not been allowed to take over.

I experienced some initial difficulty in obtaining participants for this study—not because those I approached were unwilling to take part, but because they felt they had nothing to tell me. Leg ulcers had become such a taken-for-granted part of normal living that the differences the ulcers had made to their lives were no longer immediately obvious, and were only revealed to them during the reflection involved in the interview process. At the end of an interview it was common for participants to express their surprise about how much was involved with their ulcers. Lives had continued despite the ulcers. Although Jim and Don had active ulcers for much of their adult lives, they continued to work full-time in blue-collar jobs, except for several periods when hospitalisation or complete bed rest at home was forced upon them.

Benner and Wrubel (1989, p. 136) state that 'a person with a long term illness does not simply take a temporary leave of absence from life. One is forced to let go of life as it was lived . . . [With chronic illness] life is not so much interrupted as reshaped.' The majority of the study participants were remarkably philosophical in their acceptance of their ulcer(s)—they were a fact of life which could not be ignored. The situation may not be satisfactory, but there is no choice but to accept it:

> (Do you find the loss of privacy . . .?)
>
> *Oh, I find that maddening. But I can't do anything about it. You have just got to accept it.* (Betty)

Hope of a permanent cure was common among most study participants, even though they acknowledged the chances of this happening were slight. After a period when her ulcers had been particularly troublesome, Connie needed to be able to hope for better things in the future:

> *You just keep hoping that something will work. But they can get very sore, especially when you get tired. I would hate to have these for the rest of my life.* (Connie)

Study participants who were able to do their own dressings could achieve considerable independence. Jim, for example, was unhappy with the way his ulcers had been dressed by a nurse who was not familiar with his wound management:

> *Leave it until tomorrow, and then I'll take it off. Yeah, if I find it's uncomfortable, any discomfort, I'll just take it off.*

When study participants do take control of some aspect of the management of their ulcers, they become vulnerable to accusations by health professionals that they do not want their ulcers to heal. In actual fact, control is exerted not in an attempt to prevent healing, but in response to the body aware of itself, and a sense of the need to act. Jim had extensive experience with the wound-care product used by the nurse that morning, and knew that the way it had been applied would later cause considerable discomfort once he was up and about.

Connie took charge when there was confusion about her allocation of compression stockings on discharge from hospital, refusing to accept that they did not need changing every day: 'You don't wear your stockings two days running.'

Some control must be exerted over life, even if the ulcers themselves refuse to be controlled. The body can never be trusted, but life cannot be dominated by the body's unreliability. Long-established patterns of living may need to be modified and new coping strategies developed, but over a period of time the differences created by the ulcers become part of the normal way of being-in-the-world.

IMPLICATIONS FOR NURSING PRACTICE

Many of the difficulties experienced by the participants in this study have received little attention in existing literature, but an understanding of their significance in the overall experience of living with leg ulcers is crucial to the provision of appropriate nursing care.

A review by Thomas (1989) identified the paucity of literature relating to the control of pain from leg ulcers. Frequently, the only references to pain are in terms of its potential use as a diagnostic tool to identify the aetiology of an ulcer or the presence of a wound infection. Pain from leg ulcers is rarely discussed as a problem requiring nursing action. Hofman et al. (1997) investigated the pain experienced by 94 patients with venous leg ulcers. Sixty-four per cent of their participants reported severe pain, but fewer than 40 per cent were receiving strong analgesia.

It was also clear that pain management was not satisfactory for the men and women I interviewed. All study participants experienced pain associated with their leg ulcers, with the intensity of pain ranging from general discomfort through to an almost unbearable degree of suffering. Frequently that pain appeared to be controlled poorly, with participants expressing a belief that health professionals had little idea of the extent of the pain they were experiencing.

In a study by Hamer et al. (1994) 37 per cent of 88 respondents identified pain as being the worst thing about their leg ulcer, with the authors expressing concern that this pain received little acknowledgement from healthcare workers or researchers. The study by Roe et al. (1993) of the management of leg ulcers by 146 English community nurses identified that only 55 per cent of nurses surveyed assessed their patients' experiences of pain. A crude extrapolation of the findings of these two studies would mean that more than one-third of patients considered pain the worst thing about their ulcer, yet only half of their nurses even *assess* pain.

Difficulties in complying with the instructions to rest, the precautions needed to have a shower or bath, and the discomfort associated with bandages all strongly impact on quality of life, as discussed above. Diminished quality of life is acknowledged as part of the leg ulcer experience, but the role that treatment regimens play in this diminution is seldom recognised. For some participants the impact of treatment was as significant as the symptoms generated by the wound itself. People with leg ulcers must not only learn to live with the disease process, but also with the effects of the treatment of their wounds, treatment that may well continue for months or even years.

Some of the participants in my study described how, at times, they felt unable to fully comply with the treatment prescribed for them because previous experience led them to believe that the treatment was not in their best interest. Examples were the reluctance to consent to further skin grafting when previous grafts had failed, or repeating a trial of a dressing product that had been used previously with disastrous consequences. From the patient's perspective, the possible harm from such an intervention is likely to outweigh the potential benefits.

Temporary inconvenience, when success is virtually guaranteed as a result of treatment, is a very different matter from compliance on a long-term basis, with no similar guarantees of success.

The use of compression therapy for venous ulcers is an example of a treatment which may be considered perfectly acceptable, and indeed eminently desirable, from the health professional's perspective, but which the patient finds difficult to tolerate. Study participants felt that bandages/stockings look unsightly, and assistance was often required with their application and/or removal. The bandages/stockings were also found to be uncomfortable, particularly in warmer weather. Much attention is given in the literature to alleged non-compliance in the use of compression bandaging, but less to the acceptability of this treatment to patients.

Husband (1996, p. 53) discusses what she calls the 'precarious nature' of nursing practice relating to leg ulcer management. She suggests that it is not uncommon for the medical diagnostic and management function in such cases to be delegated to nursing staff, whose preparation for this extended role is questionable. The focus on pathology and wound management also distracts nurses from their true function of 'caring for the client in a manner that is tailored to his [*sic*] individual needs and in accordance with his [*sic*] wishes' (p. 55).

Toombs (1992, p. 10) states that 'the physician and patient apprehend illness from within the context of separate worlds, each world providing its own horizon of meaning'. Comments by study participants suggest that Toombs' remark may well be applicable also to the nurse–patient relationship. When the focus of the health professional is on wound management, and the focus of the patient is on minimising the impact of what appears to be a permanent condition so he or she can get on with life, compliance can become problematic for the patient. Roberson (1992) suggests that there should be less emphasis on the issue of non-compliance, and more attention paid to assisting individuals to live well with their chronic illness and its accompanying treatment. Particularly when curative and preventive measures are likely to be long term, compromises may be needed since, despite the best efforts of all involved, these ulcers do recur (Baker et al. 1991; Moffatt et al. 1992).

Hugh described the inconvenience of his antibiotic treatment as 'a bit of a nark'. When I mentioned his comment to another participant she became quite angry, detailing the way leg ulcers had disrupted her life: 'I can tell you it's a lot more than just a bit of a nark.' The interview excerpts that have appeared in this chapter are just a small part of the stories that participants shared with me. I believe that anyone who had the opportunity to read the entire interview transcripts could not fail to be moved by the impact the ulcers have had on the lives of these people. They would realise how hard participants have tried to comply with treatment, and just how much they want their ulcers to heal permanently. And yet, as a client group, people with ulcers seem very vulnerable to criticism, particularly in relation to the issue of whether the need for continued contact with the district nurses is the reason why their ulcers fail to heal.

Given the chronic nature of these wounds and the likelihood of visits over an extended period, it is not unreasonable to expect that friendships may develop between patient and nurse. During my years as a district nurse I became very fond of some of the patients with leg ulcers with whom I had regular contact, and I regarded them as friends. But, unlike the criticism aimed at the patients, it would never be suggested to me, as a nurse, that I was deliberately delaying wounds healing to avoid losing regular contact with those patients.

Why is it that only patients are considered likely to value these friendships? Is the nurse–patient relationship an equal one, or are patients in some way thought to be inferior? Chapple (1994, p. 68) draws our attention to the special problems associated with chronic discharging wounds and how 'we simply need to constantly remind ourselves to imagine how it is for them as we deal with their dressings, and try to include them in the human race'.

Despite their leg ulcers, the study participants were leading full and meaningful lives. Some aspects of their lives were different because of the ulcers, but nevertheless they had been able to minimise the impact of their wounds, displaying considerable courage and tenacity by getting on with life. A focus on healing wounds can easily distract health professionals from recognising this courage and tenacity, and from appreciating the chronic nature of the interruptions caused by both the wounds and their treatment.

The optimum treatment regimen, the one most likely to heal the current ulcer, may well be unmanageable in the context of an ongoing life. The challenge is for health professionals, and particularly nurses, to understand the realities of life with chronic ulcers, and to work with patients to determine the treatment that will most allow life to continue, while still facilitating wound healing.

REFERENCES

Baker, S.R., Stacey, M.C., Jopp-McKay, A.G., Hoskin, S.E. & Thompson, P.J. 1991 'Epidemiology of chronic venous ulcers' *British Journal of Surgery* no. 78, pp. 864–7

Benner, P. & Wrubel, J. 1989 *The Primacy of Caring: Stress and Coping in Health and Illness* Addison-Wesley, Menlo Park, Ca.

Callam, M.J., Harper, D.R., Dale, J.J. & Ruckley, C.V. 1988 'Chronic leg ulceration: socio-economic aspects' *Scottish Medical Journal* no. 33, pp. 358–60

Chapple, J. 1994 'Assisting wound healing' *New Zealand Practice Nurse* March, pp. 65–8

Charles, H. 1995 'The impact of leg ulcers on patients' quality of life' *Professional Nurse* vol. 10, no. 9, pp. 571–2

Cullum, N. 1994 *The Nursing Management of Leg Ulcers in the Community: A Critical Review of Research* report produced for the Department of Health by the Department of Nursing, University of Liverpool, UK

Ertl, P. 1992 'How do you make your treatment decision?' *Professional Nurse* vol. 7, no. 8, pp. 543–52

Hamer, C., Cullum, N.A. & Roe, B.M. 1994 'Patients' perceptions of chronic leg ulcers' *Journal of Wound Care* vol. 3, no. 2, pp. 99–101

Hofman, D., Ryan, T.J., Arnold, F., Cherry, G.W., Lindholm, C., Bjellerup, M. & Glynn, C. 1997 'Pain in venous leg ulcers' *Journal of Wound Care* vol. 6, no. 5, pp. 222–4.

Husband, L.L. 1996 'The management of the client with a leg ulcer: precarious nursing practice' *Journal of Advanced Nursing* no. 24, pp. 53–9

Lindholm, C., Bjellerup, M., Christensen, O.B. & Zederfeldt, B. 1993 'Quality of life in chronic leg ulcer patients: an assessment according to the Nottingham Health Profile' *Acta Dermato Venerologica (Stockholm)* no. 73, pp. 440–3

Moffatt, C.J., Franks, P.J., Oldroyd, M., Bosanquet, N., Brown, P., Greenhalgh, R.M. & McCollum, C.N. 1992 'Community clinics for leg ulcers and impact on healing' *British Medical Journal* no. 305, pp. 1389–92

Nelzen, O., Bergqvist, D. & Lindhagen, A. 1994 'Venous and non-venous leg ulcers: clinical history and appearance in a population study' *British Journal of Surgery* no. 81, pp. 182–7

Roberson, M.H.B. 1992 'The meaning of compliance: patient perspectives' *Qualitative Health Research* vol. 2, no. 1, pp. 7–26

Roe, B.H., Luker, K.A., Cullum, N.A., Griffiths, J.M. & Kenrick, M. 1993 'Assessment, prevention and monitoring of chronic leg ulcers in the community: report of a survey' *Journal of Clinical Nursing* no. 2, pp. 299–306

Thomas, S. 1989 'Pain and wound management' *Community Outlook* July, pp. 11–15

Toombs, S.K. 1992 *The Meaning of Illness: A Phenomenological Account of the Different Perspectives of Physician and Patient* Kluwer, Netherlands

van Manen, M. 1990 *Researching Lived Experience: Human Science for an Action Sensitive Pedagogy* Althouse Press, London and Ontario

Wise, G. 1986 'Overcoming loneliness' *Nursing Times* vol. 82, no. 22, pp. 37–42

four

On confronting life and death

VICKI PARKER

This chapter is based on a research project carried out in a large tertiary hospital in New South Wales, Australia. The design of this research project involved a clinical field study using triangulation of data sources, including participant observation, review of the patients' notes within the intensive care unit (ICU) and interviews with patients following their discharge from ICU. The five men and five women who participated in the study ranged in age from 17 to 75 and were admitted to ICU for a variety of emergency reasons. As a result the patients were not in any way prepared for what they experienced.

The motivation for this study came from the author's twelve years of experience as a critical care nurse.

SINCE THE INCEPTION of the intensive care unit (ICU) over 30 years ago, there has been interest in the effects of the highly technologised environment on those who receive intensive care. In response, there is a growing body of literature directed towards understanding patients' experiences in ICU. The earlier of these works, appearing in the late 1960s, focused on what was observed by physicians and nurses (Kornfeld 1969; McKegney 1966), rather than drawing on patients' own experiences. Many subsequent studies, particularly those conducted during the 1980s, focused on the identification of stressors confronting patients in ICU (Baker 1984; Chyun 1989; Cochran & Ganong 1989; Gries & Fernsler 1988; Kleck 1984; Simpson et al. 1989; Wilson 1987). Although this approach is problematic because it focuses on the negative rather than the positive aspects of the experience, it constitutes the main body of literature directed towards understanding patients' experiences of ICU. Stressors consistently identified include pain, sleeplessness, noise, bright lights, the inability to communicate, confusion, distressing memories, dreams, hallucinations, fear, anxiety, uncertainty and technology. While there is some agreement among these studies in relation to the nature of the stressors identified, there is discrepancy as to the extent to which each stressor is considered to be a problem.

In spite of the large number of studies of this nature, very little has changed in relation to patients' reports of these aspects of their experience. This failure could be attributed to the adoption of a view of stress as resulting from the environmental or physical aspects that give rise to a problem for the patient, rather than as the meaning of the interaction the patient has with others, 'when that meaning conveys challenge, loss, threat or harm' (Benner & Wrubel 1989, p. 59). Studies examining stressors fail to identify successful management strategies patients have employed in order to cope with their ordeal. Furthermore, they do not usually consider the participation of the patient in coping, enduring and managing their own experience.

More recently, qualitative approaches have explored the meaning that critical illness has for patients and identified the various strategies patients adopt in order to deal with their experiences (Hafsteindottir 1996; Jablonski 1994; Laitinen 1996; Morse & O'Brien 1995). However, there are relatively few studies of this nature, and there still appears to be no definition of critical illness other than that which focuses on the physical threat and proximity to death.

Holloway (1993, p. 3), for instance, suggests that central to ICU nursing practice is the critically ill patient, characterised by 'the presence of, or being at risk for developing life threatening problems'. The concept of critical illness itself is not examined. Rather the assumption seems to be that critical illness differs from other illness only in a quantitative sense—its speed of onset or degree of physiological disruption. However comprehensive the approach adopted by critical-care nursing texts, what is missing is any sense of the person whose life is threatened and whose emotional, psychological or social integrity is at risk. For the purposes of this study, critical illness is defined in line with Kleinman (1988) and Benner and Wrubel (1989), who understand illness as primarily existential, a lived experience which affects the person as a whole.

During the twelve years I worked as a nurse in ICU there were many occasions where it was impossible for me to ask patients how they were feeling or what they required to help lessen their suffering, or to help them cope with their situations. Daily I experienced the frustration and difficulty of trying to communicate effectively with patients, and of having to provide care while not being entirely sure of their needs and wishes. It was this lack of knowing and the need to better understand patients' experiences that provided the impetus for this study. Through examination of personal experiences, this chapter highlights critical illness as not only physically and emotionally life threatening, but also as significantly affecting every aspect of a person's existence.

THE EXPERIENCE OF BEING CRITICALLY ILL IN ICU

The ten participants in this study came to ICU unprepared and without choice. Their state of health was such that they had no options. Finding themselves in an alien environment, their lives had been completely disrupted. They felt helpless and dependent on others. They suffered physical pain and discomfort, fear of the unknown and fear of death. As one participant said, 'it was not a nice place to be'.

Unnaturalness and disruption

The most obvious, and perhaps the most important, aspect of experiencing ICU as a patient is the total unnaturalness of the situation. Nothing is normal. The environment is unfamiliar, as is the life patients are forced to live within it:

> *I can remember waking up down there and I had no idea where I was and why I was in pain and I couldn't remember a thing of what had happened or why I was there or anything else. One of the nurses said to me, 'Oh you know, you are in hospital' and so forth, and then it sort of came back and it was really depressing for me because I was about the only conscious person in Intensive Care. I was opposite this old man and he had tubes and everything coming out of him, and every so often they were putting down, it was like a long plastic thing, it looked like a condom that was going down and I didn't know what they were doing and it was to clear him out or something cos they did the same to me. I*

thought it was really depressing, and I don't know how anyone can work up there. The doctors come around and they all stand outside and they talk about you but they don't actually tell you what they are saying and you pick up little bits and pieces and sometimes it sounds worse than what it probably is or whatever. I didn't think I was going to get out of there that time and I really thought I was [going to die]. It's just the not knowing what is going on around you and all, just sickness, and everywhere you go there are sick people. (Mary)

The sudden and immediate nature of the disruption to their lives was reflected in the way the patients experienced consciousness, time, embodiment and uncertainty, not just in the early hours of admission, but throughout the entire time they spent in ICU. Critical illness is essentially and overwhelmingly disruptive. The pervasive nature of disruption was evident in participants' responses to altered and changing states of consciousness, where often they 'awoke' to new realisations of bodily restraint, incapacity and uncertainty. Rather than getting used to their situation, as the patients drifted between states of consciousness they encountered 'new realities' each time they awoke. In this way critical illness and injury induced temporal dislocation and patients lost a sense of the flow of time. Unable to use their time, patients lost track of it.

Everyone in the study described losing days, having a gap in their memory where some days cannot be accounted for. Some lost as few as two or three days, others up to seventeen. Loss of days resulted in an inability to continue life based on complete knowledge of their past and a difficulty in predicting and anticipating the future. Part of their life was lost to them and they could never go back to retrieve it. Melissa, who had no memory of her accident or of being in ICU at all, tried to explain it:

So much doesn't make any sense, it's weird, to suddenly wake up like this [badly injured] and not know how you got here. It's frustrating because you need to get on with your life.

Melissa lost not only the days that she had spent in ICU, but also a week of her life prior to her accident. The insecurity resulting from this type of temporal displacement dismantles established connections to the world.

Displacement and disablement

Feelings of dislocation from the world were amplified by restriction in movement, loss of speech and participants' inability to purposefully direct themselves physically into the world and respond to its challenges. For most participants, the initial realisation of their dire predicament involved experiencing their body's failure to respond in its usual and expected way. They told of how they awoke to find they were unable to talk, move or respond as they usually would. They found themselves trapped in a body that was still able to hear, see, feel and interpret the world but unable to physically react to events occurring around them and to them.

Disablement meant that the patients experienced their body, its disability and the world in strange and threatening ways. However, it was not just the body that was disabled; physical disablement went hand in hand with damage to the self, resulting from dislocation from a personal life, and the subsequent doubt and loss of autonomy. This damage to self is described in autobiographical writing by Moore (1991) in relation to his critical injury, and by Murphy (1987), who suffered a more insidious form of disability that eventually led to quadriplegia. Damage in both these instances was referred to not so much as physical impairment, but more as the loss of something essentially valuable and desirable—being at home with oneself in one's body.

Experienced as uncomfortable, painful or dyspnoeic, bodies and questions of physical safety were unable to be ignored. Halting of bodily rhythm confined the person's consciousness to the present time and immediate concerns, particularly the possibility of death. Not only did participants experience the inability to behave as expected, but they often became aware of strange bodily experiences and of bodily functions, such as breathing, that had previously been invisible and taken for granted.

This foregrounding of that which had previously been invisible in some cases superseded awareness of any damage to their bodies. Several participants were unaware of injuries or operations, sometimes for almost the whole of the time they spent in ICU. Even though they could see signs of damage, such as blood, stitches, swelling and bruising, they were able to dissociate themselves from the physical appearance of their bodies. Rather, the focus of their concern was the disabling consequences of the injury, the absence of a body that acted for them and as them. Only when they were the source of unrelieved pain were injuries or wounds apparent to conscious awareness. In some cases this was of real concern to nurses because it meant that patients behaved with little regard for their injuries, attempting to get out of bed or roll over, as well as other behaviours that were potentially damaging.

Ambiguity and uncertainty

Experiences of being critically ill in ICU were affected by altered perceptual acuity and the inability to clarify perceptions and ideas. This meant that participants lived with the unknown and the imagined, and were often unsure and confused. Often these factors came together in the creation of experiences that were neither entirely real nor completely imagined but, rather, somewhere in between. The unreal nature of situations, together with a sense of dissociation, caused participants to feel as though they existed in a kind of 'in-between world'—between life and death, imagination and reality, sleep and wakefulness, the past and the future, the known and the unknown. They reported experiencing hallucinations, dreams, nightmares and doubt.

Living with doubt and uncertainty engendered fear and insecurity and undermined the patients' ability to interpret what was happening and participate knowingly in activities occurring to and around them. Yet 'knowing' was not necessarily seen as achievable or even desirable. The patients' experience of uncertainty was ambiguous and paradoxical. They knew, or at least suspected, that they were critically ill, but they did not know why or how it came about, or what was happening and going to happen. They needed to know so that they could make sense of and gain some control over the situation and yet they did not want to know because of fear of what might be known.

Not knowing caused them to worry and at times to think the worst, which affected their ability to rest, to sleep and to concentrate on cooperating with their care. The strain of not knowing was almost unbearable, but equally unbearable was the fearful apprehension of knowing. As participants became more aware of their circumstances, new uncertainties arose. Most were concerned for the welfare of their families and what might happen if they died or were incapacitated. Participants who were awake and in ICU for a longer period were more likely to be overwhelmed by the uncertain nature of their situation.

In situations where participants perceived that they were safe, knowing what was happening was not as important and uncertainty seemed to be less threatening. Having others present, particularly family, enabled participants to feel safe in uncertain circumstances, as Ellen explained:

> *I s'pose I couldn't really work out what was true and what wasn't true you know, but when I think back now, I still think over things in my mind and I think, 'Well, did that happen or didn't it happen?' But, I*

suppose it was just part and parcel of, well, not knowing really what was happening you know. It was just that I was there, I knew I was sick and I was being well cared for and the family was there.

In this way, knowledge of the situation was constituted by personal experience, and the adage 'what you don't know can't hurt you' aptly applied. Being told what happened was not really the same as knowing what happened. Some of the participants were glad they did not know because it meant they had been saved the pain and the distress of knowingly living the experience.

A balance of known and unknown was tolerable to the study participants, but as the scales tipped towards greater uncertainty the situation became less bearable. Living in a situation where nothing was clear often transformed the unclear into terrifying possibilities. For example, Ellen feared that she was going to fall out of bed when she was held close to the edge, perceiving the distance between the bed and the floor to be ten or twelve feet rather than three or four. Similarly, staff were described as just two or three feet away by those who felt safe, and sometimes twenty or 30 feet away by those who were frightened. For some of the participants, like Phillip, being closed in and alone intensified feelings of helplessness, placing them at the mercy of their imagination:

As long as I could see something or someone it didn't bother me but when I was [closed in], they'd close the door and that's when it would worry me and it wasn't a good room for me. If I couldn't have seen anything it would have driven me mad. Like as it was, it sort of turned [on] the imagination I'd say.

Reality and confusion

The ability of participants to trust their interpretation of the world was further diminished by frequent dreams and hallucinations, and the confusion in trying to discern between them and reality. Although the circumstances and the details of experiences differed, there were consistent patterns and themes which emerged from the participants' descriptions. A particularly common theme was that of being restrained or confined. Participants told of being tied down, buried in sand and being held prisoner—situations where their bodies had lost the capacity to move and create their own space. Some suggested that drugs, fever and lack of sleep may have contributed to their strange experiences, as was the case in this story related by David:

> *Yeah, it was shocking. One night in particular, I had a bit of a fever and that, and not knowing that I had a fever, I do now. I just couldn't sleep, and I was sort of thinking, I was half asleep and the mind was playing up. I felt like I was wired on to a machine, that I had to keep breathing to keep the machine working, that if I didn't keep the machine working then the nurse was going to come in and go mad at me. Cos I was sort of half dreaming half, you know, cos of the noise of the trachy [tracheostomy] when you breathe in and out. I thought I was driving a machine and all the traction bed around, and all the tubing and that. Like I said, with the fever and that the mind does funny things, sort of hard to explain, like I thought I was driving a sheep shearing machine. I could feel pulleys and you know as I was breathing. I was like driving a bellow that was keeping stuff happening and the machine was keeping me happening and not vice versa but I couldn't sleep because I had to concentrate on keeping this machine going, but I guess I snapped out of that.*

Participants often found themselves between the two worlds of imagination and reality. In David's story above, the orthopaedic bedframe, with its pulleys and ropes, the noisy movement of air through the tracheostomy and the persistent reminders by the nurse to keep taking deep breaths, allowed the construction of a perfectly feasible, although inaccurate, situation. There were many more examples of this phenomenon.

Doubt, dreams and hallucinations increased participants' feelings of vulnerability. Being unable to ask questions and clarify their thoughts engendered feelings of helplessness and confined them within the lifespace that was available to them, a space that was characterised by sickness and the possibility of death.

BEING VOICELESS, HELPLESS AND DEPENDENT, AND CLOSE TO SICKNESS AND DEATH

Being voiceless was one of the most significant features of the participants' experience of being critically ill in ICU. Not being able to talk as a consequence of intubation or application of CPAP (continuous positive airways pressure) resulted not only in difficulty in communicating with others but also in loss of voice, literally and metaphorically, as a means by which to represent themselves and their immediate needs. Even when patients were extubated, loss of being in touch with the circumstances of their lives and a lack of knowledge of events, therapies, technology and the like excluded them from participating in decision-making and prevented them from speaking out.

Attempting to communicate while intubated was described as 'frustrating' and 'hopeless'. Not being able to speak was debilitating enough, but other forms of communication that would normally substitute for speech, such as writing and touch, were also impaired. The impossibility of speech meant that participants were often not consulted in relation to events affecting them. Assumed to be unable to speak for themselves, they were alienated and excluded. Although they were distressed by the inability to make known their needs, a significant amount of the participants' distress related to the inability to release emotional tension and gain comfort through conversation with others. Without the ability to speak, patients felt as though they were alone in a world removed from the world of others. While hearing the voices of others, particularly family, was important, patients highlighted the importance of being able to respond.

Perceiving their bodies as disabled and being unsure of the response of their bodies left participants feeling unsafe and insecure. In many instances bodies were experienced as not only disabled but also painfully, awkwardly or distressingly able. This dys-ablement was most apparent in experiences of pain and dyspnoea, which at times seemed to take them hostage and constrict their world of experience to a painfully disabled body and present. In particular, dyspnoea became the singular focus of participants' existence and, at the same time, threatened their very existence. In some cases participants suffered several overwhelming symptoms simultaneously.

The unbearable and unrelenting nature of symptoms was one of the factors that led almost all of the participants to feel that, at some time during their experience, they were going to die. Death as a strong possibility was felt to have a pervasive presence in ICU. Living with death as present was experienced by participants at different times in different ways. When patients realised where they were and how sick the people around them were, they were reminded of their own mortality. Mary, for example, felt extremely unsafe. Previously, when she had had cancer and undergone chemotherapy she had not felt that she was going to die. In ICU, however, it felt to her as though death was at hand. Feeling very sick, not being able to breathe and not being reassured that she would live, caused her to believe that she could not be saved, that she was beyond help. The urgency of the situation and the feeling of impending doom made her ICU experience very different from her experience of cancer, where death was a possible prognosis rather than an imminent and pervasive possibility.

Interestingly, a number of participants experienced a sense of the presence, in one form or another, of dead family members or friends. This phenomenon was usually manifested in dreams or in a kind of 'sensing'. Mary reported hearing her mother's footsteps and anticipated her arrival, even though she knew her mother had died several years earlier. Veronica dreamed of dead neighbours, friends and relatives every night, even after she had been discharged from hospital. Some of the study participants who described such incidents were not always frightened or even surprised by their experiences, just puzzled as to how they occurred. For others, especially Veronica whose dreams of dead people persisted, the experience was profoundly disturbing.

Sometimes it was the overwhelming and oppressive nature of their present circumstances that made participants think that they would die. At other times the feeling was not so much that of impending doom, but rather of what seemed like a logical assumption that death must be near. Laura explained how she felt:

> *All the family started coming in droves and I thought, 'Am I really sick, what is everyone doing here?' and then a friend of mine sent in a priest to see me and I thought, 'You are not giving me the last rites are you?' Many a time I thought I wouldn't make it. Things just seemed to be getting worse and worse with tubes down my nose and I couldn't eat or anything. I couldn't hold things down. And the blood clot, that really upset me most of all and I did say to Mum, 'Am I going to get out of here alive?' Yeah, I was so frightened.*

Living with a sense of death-as-near created feelings of fear and panic. Not wanting to die, participants struggled to survive, and this struggle meant mustering the strength to continue to deal with hardship and adversity, and to maintain the will to live.

STRUGGLING TO SURVIVE

The threat of death saw the participants call into action all the physical and emotional forces they could employ in the defence of their personal safety. A struggle was mounted on the basis of experiencing fear, panic, pain and dyspnoea. The threat of death was felt to be stronger at some times than at others and was driven by the perception of and the accompanying meaning associated with various events that occurred during ICU hospitalisation, including being turned, suctioned or manacled. Responses to threat were multidimensional, intricate and personalised. Reacting to threat involved the mobilisation of instinctive, primordial responses, with participants becoming personally involved in a struggle for their own life and investing their time and energy to maintain vigilance.

In the face of perceived threat, when patients panicked, they seemed to have incredible physical strength. Several cases were observed during the study of participants reacting violently, attempting to get out of bed, pulling out tubes and lashing out at staff. Terror and fear appeared to capture the patients' bodies and intentions, their determination and commitment evident in their bulging eyes, contorted grimaces and tense and primed muscles. In some cases it took four or five people to hold a person down. Some participants had no memory of these incidents, while others were able to describe the panic or horrifying hallucinations that precipitated their behaviour.

Robert, at 75 and usually physically debilitated by emphysema, managed to kick and thrash violently in his efforts to repel five people who were attempting to restrain him. Knowing that they were trying to save his life did not make any difference. Struggling to get the mask off his face and pulling out the endotracheal tube were actions over which he felt he had no control:

> *Apparently I had pulled the tube out and I can't recall that part, that I'd do that. I must have been looking for air to do a thing like that. I suppose to me in my semi-delirious state I was more or less thinking, 'I've got to get the airways clear.'*

Reacting in this way seemed to be unrelated to conscious appreciation of the situation, with some participants puzzled by their apparent lack of regard for their own safety. At other times, participants reported how they had committed themselves to survival and became actively involved in ensuring their own safety. Living inside a body under threat mandated patients' commitment to its continued existence. This interest, however, was threatened by the corrosive nature of persistent pain or dyspnoea and the de-energising power of the unknown.

Participants expressed how at times they did not care whether they lived or died. Being alive was just too difficult and a future of continued dyspnoea or pain was felt to be beyond enduring:

> *I didn't care . . . all I know is I felt terrible and they were going to give me something to put me to sleep and I wished they would hurry up and do that. One thought passed my mind, 'What if they put me on this, they called it the breathing machine and I didn't wake up?' and I really didn't care at that stage. I just wanted to be asleep so I*

> *didn't feel. And mainly I was frightened because I couldn't breathe . . . I just wanted to be asleep so I didn't know one way or the other. I just wished they would hurry up and do it.* (Mary)

But not caring to live because the struggle was felt to be too difficult to endure was in hindsight not really a wish to die but rather a wish for reprieve; to be free of pain or dyspnoea, or simply to be allowed to rest. Struggle involved overcoming or at least enduring what at times seemed like overwhelming physical and emotional hardship:

> *Suffocating and not being able to breathe was what scared me the most I think. The more that I thought about it the worse I got. If I could have not been so scared I probably would not have had to be on the ventilator. I thought I was going to die because I couldn't breathe properly.* (Mary)

The struggle was both physical and emotional. Phillip was in ICU for over a month and saw many patients come and go. The prompt recovery of other patients emphasised his own failure to recover and reinforced his feelings that he would eventually die. The longer it went on, the harder it was for him to believe he would 'make it'. At times the only way out seemed death:

> *Well I was starting to wonder, seeing them all move and everyone was bloody going and I wasn't, you know. I did seem to think I'd never get out. And I had a few nightmares, you know, but ah they weren't real good . . . I thought I was in a box [coffin] a couple of times and then I thought, 'bugger this I'm not going [to die]', but then I thought 'Christ, what's the use of it', and then I'd think 'if you keep thinking like this you will die'. So, it got me like that and a couple of times, it was pretty hard.*

Many of the participants vacillated between despondency and determination, and they had to work hard to muster the energy to keep fighting. Commitment to survival meant that participants devised strategies by which they could maintain some control over their situation. This often involved becoming vigilant about the events and activities happening around them. Becoming vigilant involved being acutely aware of the circumstances surrounding their condition—staff, technology, procedures and routines—and monitoring the course of events. Vigilance was manifested in activities such as continual watching of monitors; watching of staff to see what they were doing and if they were paying attention; needing to have the door open, checking the time to see how long before treatments and procedures; and checking and caring for lines, ensuring that they were attached and that they were not lying on them. While being vigilant increased patients' capacity to know what was happening around them, it resulted in lack of sleep, and panic reduced their ability to interpret situations and respond positively.

When suffering or doubt became unbearable, vigilance was unsustainable. Most of the participants came to realise that they were incapable of managing their situation. Although they had mounted their own battle for life, they could not do it alone. Generally God, family members and staff were seen to be responsible co-custodians and co-carers although this depended on the person, their circumstances and their beliefs.

CRITICAL ILLNESS AS SHARED EXPERIENCE

The importance of being with others in ICU was demonstrated most clearly by the participants' fear of being alone. The presence of others was experienced as possibly the most important element in making the experience bearable for participants. It confirmed their existence and allowed them to feel that others were there with them and for them. But even when there were many people around, participants sometimes felt ignored and vulnerable. In turn, the perception of being alone was intensified by feelings of vulnerability and fear.

In an environment filled with that which was unknown and uncertain, recognising others and being recognised was felt to be paramount. While being with someone was better than being alone, being with those who knew and loved them provided participants with a sense of constancy and security.

The importance of family

Critical illness was seen to be the business of the family; it involved only those who were intimately connected with each other. There was no room for well-meant but casual concern. It was a time for focusing on the situation at hand, pulling together, drawing close and gathering collective strength. Where families were present and participants were not able to speak or act on their own behalf, responsibility was automatically and unquestioningly transferred to the family.

In the initial period of ICU hospitalisation participants and their families were afraid that they may lose each other and they were concerned about each other's welfare. It was upsetting for participants to know that they were the cause of pain and suffering to those who loved them, while they themselves were powerless to do anything about it. Knowing that their families were there was comforting, but it was also difficult to witness their distress and to not be able to reach out to them. Veronica was extremely close to her two daughters who were with her constantly:

> *I can remember my daughter and the doctor putting his arm around her. I don't know why she was crying. I guess I do, but the actual reason I don't know . . . it was very difficult.*

Families and loved ones provided a sense of home for participants, a safe, certain and predictable shelter in an otherwise hostile world. Their presence was possibly the only thing that could be guaranteed.

Several of the participants became upset when they talked about their family's contribution to their experience. The importance of having their family with them and the magnitude of the emotion this evoked defied easy description, either because they could not find the words or they were too overcome to speak at all. Participants often knew that they were important to their families, but for many, critical illness brought out with new insight the emotional strength and commitment that bound families together. When threatened by the possible loss of each other, the participants and their families demonstrated that commitment:

> *Whereas before they would always give you a kiss and a hug, but never actually come out and say how much you mean to them. I know what I mean to them but they never actually tell you, you know. But this last fortnight they've told me. The staff did a wonderful job, but the boys and Amy [daughter], their moral support . . . If I didn't have them I think it might have been a different kettle of fish. Like nothing was too much trouble, the boys lifted me and Amy fed me.* (Ellen)

Critical illness as a new and difficult experience elicited the expression of personal attributes and behaviours that may not have been evident in previous experiences. Family members came to know more about each other, and themselves and their individual and collective capabilities. Nearly all the participants spoke of their family being drawn closer together by the experience. In this way, critical illness, although extremely difficult to bear, also confirmed and strengthened important relationships. Established and intimate relationships allowed for the infusion of faith and love that was not available, at least not in the same dimensions, from any other source. Participants believed this emotional and spiritual sustenance was just as important, or perhaps even more important, than the lifesaving strategies employed by medical and nursing staff.

The events surrounding the experience of critical illness were often remembered not as the singular memory of one person but as the combined memory of the family constructed from telling and retelling the story together. There were events that happened during the time that participants were in ICU of which they were not aware. Having been present throughout the experience, family members were able to fill in the gaps for the patient, locating events in time and chronicling the experience. In talking about the experience, patients and their families construct a collective memory of events, with participants sometimes not sure if they remembered the experience or remembered being told about it. This sharing helped solidify the memory and give meaning to the experience. In contrast, the one participant who had no family and very few visitors came to doubt his own memories and had no-one with whom to confirm his experience retrospectively. In the absence of family, nurses were often the only people who could provide valuable information to patients about their experience.

Encounters with staff

'If it hadn't been for them' was a phrase used by almost all the participants in reference to staff. They all felt that without the expert care of nurses and doctors they would not be alive, and they continually expressed their admiration and gratitude. Feeling indebted often coloured patients' perceptions of staff, and participants were reluctant to share experiences that reflected badly on those who had been instrumental in saving their life. Even so, very few of the participants remembered individual nurses' or doctors' names, and they knew nothing about the personal lives of the people who cared for them. Those that were remembered were most often remembered for their competence, kindness, empathy and diligence.

It was not just that the staff were perceived to be good at the technical aspects of their job; participants were confident with them only when they were genuinely committed to their patients. This commitment was demonstrated through being close and being involved with the person and his or her situation. Being involved meant being attuned to people's needs—seeing, hearing and being together with them as they faced their fears and suffered pain and anguish. For Mary (who suffered respiratory failure and sepsis), it was the coaching and the constant reassurance of staff that helped her cope. Even though she still panicked, she felt it would have been much worse if it had not been for the nurse who helped her through the terrifying moments when she struggled to breathe. Mostly, however, it was the nurses' appreciation and anticipation of participants' needs and sensitivity to their emotional frailty that made the difference. The difference between descriptions of caring and uncaring encounters was characterised by presence, closeness and involvement, as opposed to absence, distance and disinterest.

Participants described how they became concerned and angry with staff who did not inspire trust or who failed to demonstrate caring or appropriate regard for them. Developing trust, however, often took time and became a real problem when each day a different nurse was assigned to care for them. The demeanour of staff was also seen to be important in creating a comfortable atmosphere. Staff who did not smile and talk with participants, or who were preoccupied with the technical aspects of their work were perceived as indifferent.

A further aspect of the encounter with staff was the contrast between intimacy and indifference. In the participants' descriptions of caring encounters it is the intimacy of the relationship that seems most important with nurses occupying the same space the same moment, as participants, touching and reassuring them. These very personal and intimate encounters stood out in contrast to the busy technical world of ICU, where faces and forms blurred as staff rushed by. The former is a situation of sensitivity and affirmation, the latter of insensitivity and alienation. This contrast was made more striking by the lack of middle-ground encounters, where nurses and participants could share time, conversations and some detail of each other's lives. Lack of reciprocity was what made participants feel like 'just a patient'.

As participants began to recover and became more aware of their own needs, they also became aware of their inability to fend for themselves and therefore their dependence on others. For some patients this recognition resulted in their feeling depressed and vulnerable. Yet, at the same time, the amount of attention they received from staff was likely to be reduced as they were perceived to be stable and so not requiring constant surveillance. Staff were likely to be busy with other more seriously ill patients, perhaps too busy to recognise the patients' emotional needs or to provide them with support. Some patients felt that nurses were more concerned with preventing death than with caring for the living. Not that any of the participants felt that this should not be so—but the reduced attention did not lessen their needs or the sense of fragility they felt as they came to realise what they had been through. When participants felt vulnerable and emotionally fragile, it helped if staff acknowledged their patients' feelings and interpreted these feelings as natural human responses to a threatening predicament.

Emotional fragility was one source of personal vulnerability for patients in ICU. Managing the inadequate and undisciplined body exposed to others was another. While in ICU, participants were unclothed and deprived of means by which they could maintain privacy and control of their intimate bodily functions. Being unable to attend to personal cleanliness was a great source of embarrassment and the ultimate form of dependence on others. Participants often felt apologetic for making a mess even though they knew they could not help it. They were affronted and embarrassed by the need for others to not only witness the inadequacies their bodies presented, but also to clean their bodies in a way that no-one had done since they were young children. In not making an issue of the situation, staff were able to reduce the embarrassment and humiliation that threatened to take over relationships.

Staff were seen as special because they were able to control their responses to the smell and sight of bodily waste, and to unself-consciously tend to the removal of faeces and sputum, cleaning participants' bodies, changing their bed linen and making them feel clean and comfortable. Participants were extremely grateful for these ministrations and stressed the significance of being washed and clean as fundamental to feeling cared for.

Being faced with critical illness

Knowing that staff were busy with other patients whose condition was more critical than their own made participants feel insignificant, a feeling that was reinforced by the sight of other critically ill patients and their upset and vigilant families:

> *I could see them trying to move different parts of his body, he did have a tube in his throat, he was probably on that ventilator. I could certainly see he wasn't conscious or doing anything.* (Mary)

When viewing other critically ill patients, what participants usually saw was a body. They often could not tell if the person was male or female or what was wrong with them, or if they were conscious or even alive. They were bodies, moved but not moving, attached to machines with tubes inserted, lying there still and silent, disconnected from the world and the impact this had on suffering families. The sight of others struck lifeless illuminated for participants human frailty and vulnerability. It was the inability to step aside from the experiences of others that was most painful for participants—being unable to escape meant that they were forced to witness the experiences of those around them. Mary, the mother of three young boys, recounted the distress she felt seeing a critically ill child:

> *I couldn't help getting involved in it. I guess because she was little and I've got a six-year-old. And she just lay there for weeks and weeks and there was no progress, no nothing, how awful.*

Patients in ICU could not witness the suffering of others as disinterested observers, and they were inexorably drawn into the experiences of their fellow patients. In identifying with others and their predicament, participants questioned their own safety. They often saw themselves as better off than others, since they had come through the worst of it, whereas others might not. Feeling lucky and extremely grateful, participants reflected on their experience and were glad to escape ICU with their lives.

The proximity of death

In dealing with and trying to come to terms with what they had been through, participants questioned, reflected, puzzled over and forgot aspects of their experience. Having 'nearly died' raised for participants questions about their life and their death. They wondered why they had survived and what their death would have meant. In many ways their previous life, which had perhaps seemed ordinary, took on new meaning and was viewed with a clearer perspective and greater appreciation. Participants described how they now realised what their families meant to them and what it meant to be alive. This metamorphosis was characterised not only by mindful appreciation and transformed perspective, but also by an awakening of bodily perception and appreciation of the world. Their experience had shaken the very foundations on which their lives had been lived prior to their experience of critical illness. Essentially, every aspect of their existence had been disrupted. The following poem, derived from Ellen's story, captures the essence of what surviving a critical illness meant for her:

Oh, it's been an experience all right,
  a real experience.
    I nearly died, you know.
The kids were all there with me,
  they were so good.
They told me 'I love you Mum'.

I nearly died you know.
The nurses were great,
I wasn't really scared.
I thought 'It'll be okay if someone is here'.
I nearly died, you know.
The doctor came one morning,
he stood at the end of my bed and smiled,
I didn't know who he was. He said,
'I saved your life, you know'.
Ah, we laugh about it now,
it wasn't so bad.
It's all in the past, behind me now.
I nearly died you know.
The Sallies came on Sunday,
they sang a few songs.
And I cried like a baby.
Oh God,
I nearly died, you know.

CONCLUSION

The experience of having been critically ill in ICU is essentially a human encounter, characterised by inconsistency, paradox and ambiguity. In journeying to the edge, the participants in this study were tormented, challenged, displaced and disabled. Their experiences were fundamentally embodied and relational. The disruption to their lives was almost complete and yet they emerged intact and in some ways renewed and fortified. They struggled to survive, to maintain a sense of themselves and to overcome hardship. The importance of families in helping them achieve these cannot be overemphasised. They told their stories in order to make less traumatic the experiences of others who may become critically ill and be admitted to ICU.

It is essential that nurses and others who care for the critically ill understand the nature of their experience. For without insightful appreciation, we are at risk of underestimating the extent of the disruption and the overwhelming emotional and physical hardship patients face. We need to be ever vigilant and sensitive to the needs of both patients and their all-important families. This means transcending the technical culture and environment of ICU; seeing and responding to human frailty and vulnerability; and recognising and fortifying both individual strengths and capacities, as well as collective support systems. I hope that this study's findings will generate further interest and research, challenge nurses to question their practice, and ensure patients and families are always the central focus of intensive care nursing.

REFERENCES

Baker, C.F. 1984 'Sensory overload and noise in the ICU: sources of environmental stress' *Critical Care Quarterly* vol. 6, pp. 66–79

Benner, P. & Wrubel, J. 1989 *The Primacy of Caring. Stress and Coping in Illness and Health* Addison-Wesley, Menlo Park, Ca.

Chyun, D. 1989 'Patients' perceptions of stressors in intensive care and coronary care units' *Focus on Critical Care* vol. 16, pp. 206–11

Cochran, J. & Ganong, L.H. 1989 'A comparison of nurses' and patients' perceptions of intensive care unit stressors' *Journal of Advanced Nursing* vol. 14, pp. 1038–43.

Gries, M. & Fernsler, J. 1988 'Patients' perceptions of the mechanical ventilation experience' *Focus on Critical Care* vol. 15, no. 2, pp. 52–8

Hafsteindottir, T.B. 1996 'Patients' experiences of communication during the respirator treatment period' *Intensive and Critical Care Nursing* vol. 12, pp. 261–71

Holloway, N. 1993 *Nursing the Critically Ill Adult* Addison-Wesley, Menlo Park, Ca.

Jablonski, R. 1994 'The experience of being mechanically ventilated' *Qualitative Health Research* vol. 4, no. 2, pp. 186–207

Kleck, H.G. 1984 'ICU Syndrome: onset, manifestations, treatment, stressors and prevention' *Critical Care Quarterly* vol. 6, no. 4, pp. 21–8

Kleinman, A. 1988 *The Illness Narratives. Suffering, Healing and the Human Condition* Basic Books, New York

Kornfeld, D.S. 1965 'The hospital environment: its impact on the patient' *Stress and Survival. The Emotional Realities of Life Threatening Illness* ed. C. Garfield, Mosby, St Louis

——1969 'Psychiatric view of the intensive care unit' *British Medical Journal* vol. 1, pp. 108–10

——1971 'Psychiatric problems of an intensive care unit' *Medical Clinics of North America* vol. 55, no. 5, pp. 1353–63

Laitinen, H. 1996 'Patients' experience of confusion in the intensive care unit following cardiac surgery' *Intensive and Critical Care Nursing* vol. 12, pp. 79–83

McKegney, F.P. 1966 'The intensive care syndrome. The definition, treatment and prevention of a new "disease of medical progress"' *Connecticut Medicine* vol. 30, no. 9, pp. 633–6

Moore, A.R. 1991 *Cry of the Damaged Man* Penguin, Melbourne

Morse, J.M. & O'Brien, B. 1995 'Preserving self: from victim to patient, to disabled person' *Journal of Advanced Nursing* vol. 21, pp. 886–96

Murphy, R.F. 1987 *The Body Silent* Henry Holt, New York

Simpson, T., Armstrong, S. & Mitchell, P. 1989 'Critical care management. American Association of Critical Care Nurses Demonstration Project: Patients' recollections of critical care' *Heart and Lung* vol. 18, no. 4, pp. 325–31

Wilson, V. 1987 'Identification of stressors related to patients' psychological response to the surgical intensive care' *Heart and Lung* vol. 16, no. 3, pp. 267–73 *five*

On surviving breast cancer and mastectomy

KYUNG-RIM SHIN

Kyung-Rim Shin has a longstanding interest in women's health, particularly Korean women. In her doctoral dissertation she examined correlates of depressive symptomatology in Korean–American women living in New York city. Over the past five years she has moved towards more qualitative approaches to research—a novel and challenging field for nurse academics in Korea. The study which provided the basis for this chapter is an example of such research.

PERSONAL EXPERIENCES CAN lead researchers to choose particular topics for future inquiries and to reflect more deeply on the experiences of others. They can also lead to a great sense of identification and shared understanding with research participants whose stories bring to life personal experiences which might have been forgotten or set aside. Such shared recollections touch the core of one's understanding of what it is to be a woman, to be ill and to be facing life with a new sense of uncertainty. What the present study reawakened for me was the memory of major illness and surgery—the experience of a deep sense of loss, of deprivation, beyond easy description.

On a day soon after I had completed my doctoral studies—and as a good and faithful middle-aged woman feeling satisfied with my life's achievements, personally, domestically and economically—my doctor informed me that I needed to undergo a hysterectomy. When I heard that the operation had to be performed as soon as possible, I took it to mean the end of my life was near and I was reduced to constant tears. I prepared for the operation while recollecting my life up to that time. During the week before surgery, I found myself in the hospital, full of theoretical knowledge as a nurse, but without experience to make sense of what was happening to me. During that week, I did some reflective writing about my life. Delivered to the operating room on a trolley, I felt that I would suffocate from anaesthesia and experienced severe dyspnoea. Following the operation, I faced premature menopause as a shock brought on by the sudden imbalance of hormones and the appearance of 'hot flushes'. Feeling a tightness in my chest and with a flushed face, I could not fall asleep even with the window open. My usually positive attitude towards life had been replaced with a multitude of uncertainties. I was suddenly cautious not to commit sins by means of mind, body or speech. Nowadays, when I recall this experience, I remember feeling that my whole way of life had changed.

Reflecting on my past experiences, as a nurse and as a woman, has led to my interest in the experiences of other middle-aged women, particularly those who have had a mastectomy, those who have lost one of the intrinsic parts of their body. Seeing my best friend's concern about regular tests and treatment since her mother and aunt died of breast cancer intensified the personal interest. I wrote about these experiences in my diary, which I kept throughout the study. Other influences came from reflections on literature, film and portrayals encountered in the general media—often shared during interviews by the women who took part in the study.

CULTURAL CONTEXT OF THE STUDY

There are two important contextual issues that come to light through the study of the Korean women's experience of breast cancer and mastectomy. One is that breast cancer most often affects middle-aged women, reflected in the age of the study participants who were in their 40s or early 50s. The second issue is the cultural context of the study, that of South Korea—a society coming to terms with the growing impact of Western culture, including the influences of Christian religion and Western medicine on its strongly Buddhist and Confucian values, and on its traditional social roles and health-related practices. The experience of life-threatening illness, particularly for middle-aged women, is strongly influenced by these factors, not only because those who are currently middle-aged are still of the generation brought up with a strong sense of traditional Korean culture, but also because women's roles have changed more slowly than those of men. As discussed later in this chapter, breast cancer challenges this already uncertain personal and social identity, and place of Korean middle-aged women. While the specific causes of breast cancer are not fully understood, it is relevant to note that relatively recent social developments—such as changes in diet towards a greater intake of saturated fat and high-calorie foods, and deferral of pregnancy and breast feeding (or their avoidance altogether)—have been identified as contributing factors (Oh 1993). Even at this basic biological level the experience can be seen to be both culturally bound and yet, in some ways, also universal.

The findings presented in this chapter relate to the experiences of six women, residing in a regional city in South Korea. All were interviewed twice, in tape-recorded interviews that ranged from one to four hours in length, during the period from February 1994 to February 1995. Additional data came from written descriptions provided by some of the participants. Each participant was also asked to talk of any examples of artistic representation (pictures, poems, film) that reminded or assisted them in their description of their mastectomy experience.

The views about middle age expressed by the women who participated in the study matched those reflected in Korean poetry and other literature. They acknowledged the inevitable march of time, the visible ageing seen in facial wrinkles and loss of prettiness, and the expectation that women's interests would focus on development of wisdom and virtue (Kim 1993). As in an essay by Lindberg (1959) in which women are likened to oysters destined to produce a pearl, women in the study recognised that they were expected to give of themselves, shaking off their personal ambitions, needs and desires in order to contribute to others' success and fulfilment. There is an expectation within the Korean culture that by middle age women will have learned to be generous with their time and energies for the benefit of their men, their children and their communities.

Women's breasts also, particularly in the Eastern, Buddhist tradition, represent giving, generosity and mercy. The antefixes in a traditional tiled roof protrude like nipples, and nipples are fixed on the eaves of Buddhist temples and on temple bells. Such representations of the female breast are said to symbolise the mercy of Buddha (Cho 1991). For Korean women in particular, breasts represent fertility, nurture and generous giving as they are related primarily to the function of breast feeding.

According to Korean folklore, breasts also represent food from nature—manna from heaven—and when seen in a dream are taken as portents of good. There is a story, for example, of an auspicious dream that involves a tortoise sucking a human breast. It is interpreted as a very fortunate dream, suggesting a resolution to any existing problem or a sign of meeting a helpful person (Yeo Sung Dong Ah 1995). Breasts also represent the miraculous, since as soon as a baby emerges from its mother's womb, milk which has not existed before suddenly flows (Da Jong Kyung 1995). As may be expected therefore, in traditional Oriental art breasts are represented as full and hemispherical—the shape seen by a suckling baby. When linked to the image of Buddha such breasts represent the Goddess of Mercy, again symbolising the nurturing role.

The trend in modern Korean art, however, is to represent the breast in a conical form, revealing a change towards the Western view that portrays women as sexual objects and breasts as erotic rather than nurturing organs. This change away from traditional values and representations, which disregards the actual shape of the breasts of most Korean women, has been said to show that Koreans are pursuing Western ideals and are beginning to subscribe to Western cultural values of materialism and pursuit of pleasure, discarding the long-held Confucian value of temperance (Cho 1991). It is the lack of temperance that leads to illness.

According to traditional teachings (*Dong Eu Bo Gam* 1610), breast cancer arises from a mind that is too anxious or too angry. It is said that when women endure prolonged anxiety or anger, a lump appears in the breast which becomes purplish-black on the surface. Inside the breast, however, the lump decays over a period of five to seven years with no signs of aching or itching. These are the symptoms of breast cancer.

Whatever the traditional views, most Korean women today resort to Western medicine once cancer is diagnosed, and mastectomy is the most common treatment. Several of the women who participated in the study identified strongly with the main protagonist of a recently published short story, *Rain, Rain, Rain* (Kim 1994), in which the writer describes his wife's experience of mastectomy and eventual death from metastatic cancer. The following excerpt from the story captures the sense of the uneasy co-existence of traditional and modern views and the personal sense of helplessness in the face of suffering and unavoidable death:

> She was a woman but not a woman. The hard rib could be felt under the horrible scar as if it were burnt with a hot iron. When going out, she wore an artificial breast made of silicone imported from France. How could I express my fear of the difference in touch between a real breast and a false breast? [After the mastectomy] I had wanted to have her treated with palliative care—anti-cancer medicine or radiotherapy. But people said that she would recover better through diet and traditional medicine, and warned me not to give her any more afflicting treatment after she had just undergone a painful operation. As for me, I felt pity for her as a woman. I listened to their advice because I wasn't able to make her endure any more pain or suffering. But it happened [she died] in just one year. (Kim 1994, translated here by the author)

A television drama series titled *Love and Separation*, showing on Korean television during the period I was interviewing women for my study, had an even more profound impact on the study participants. They identified closely with the lead character Sun-Ju Kim—played by a well-known writer Yang-Ja Ann—a housewife in her 40s diagnosed with breast cancer. The main themes explored in the series included a growing sense of misfortune and of doom, bargaining with God, fear of death, shock once the diagnosis of cancer was made known, reliance upon God, pain of anti-cancer therapy, reassessment of life priorities and goals, and rediscovery of being alone. The women in my study sympathised with Sun-Ju, seeing themselves in her every struggle.

Middle-aged women in Korea today are facing a crisis which goes beyond their health concerns. Many experience tensions between traditional and contemporary values and when trying to reconcile male and female roles. Middle-aged men can do what they want, hold important positions in business and society, and reach for the top. Middle-aged women do not enjoy the same privileges and many experience personal conflicts and tensions when they feel unable to gain satisfaction from the life they lead. They report feeling lonely, deprived, uneasy and dissatisfied when their marriage and family life fail to give them the sense of fulfilment they want (Choe 1992; Chung 1988; Kim 1983; Kim 1989; Yeun 1993). At the same time, when faced with the attractions and challenges of Western ideas and values, many Korean women, influenced by their upbringing, feel lost and unprepared to respond on an individual level, and internalise cultural and inter-generational conflicts. Middle-aged women in particular suffer from the traditional problem of discord with mothers-in-law, husbands and even children, all of whom expect physical care, support, and unquestioning loyalty from the woman as a daughter-in-law, wife and mother. Unable to resolve the tensions, many feel caught in situations out of their personal control and run the risk of developing health problems (Lee 1992; Shin & Park 1993).

There has been a significant increase in the incidence of breast cancer in Korea over recent years, with breast cancer occupying the third place in terms of total numbers of new cases of malignant disorders, after uterine and gastric cancer. While the incidence of uterine and gastric cancer has been decreasing, the figures for breast cancer have shown a marked increase, particularly in women over 40 years of age (Cancer Registration Office, National Medical Centre 1994). Whatever the biomedical or epidemiological explanations for this, it is not surprising that when an individual develops breast cancer traditional views about the causes of illness come to the fore.

Research studies in various countries suggest that women are at high risk of developing anxiety, mood changes and depression after a mastectomy. These feelings are often related to uncertainty about the success of surgery and the remission of cancer; less frequently they are related to a sense of femininity, cosmetic results and the reactions of husbands or partners (Ali & Khalie 1991; Chung 1991; Han 1991; Harris et al. 1991; Northouse 1989; Park 1986; Wong & Bramwell 1992). To understand more fully the experience of breast cancer and mastectomy in middle-aged Korean women, phenomenological research is needed and was employed in the study reported in this chapter.

THE EXPERIENCE OF BREAST CANCER AND MASTECTOMY

Qualitative data analysis and interpretation, using the approach detailed by van Manen (1990), resulted in the following major themes that best capture the structure of the phenomenon of having breast cancer and undergoing a mastectomy in the Korean context:

- accidental discovery of the sickness;
- searching for the cause;
- fear of separation from family and present life;
- loss of one's habitual being after mastectomy;
- drawing on others' support;
- changing attitudes to life and its priorities;
- rediscovering the importance of personal health;
- recognising that one is ultimately alone;
- learning to live in the shadow of death.

According to van Manen (1990, p. 91):

> Phenomenological themes are not objects or generalisations; metaphorically speaking they are more like knots in the webs of our experiences, around which certain lived experiences are spun and thus lived through as meaningful wholes. Themes are the stars that make up the universes of meaning we live through.

The themes in this study also form a web of interconnections of experiences rather than a chronological sequence of events. The accuracy of my interpretations was validated in a discussion with participants, who saw their individual lives and experiences captured in the web of thematic description which occupies the remainder of this chapter.

Accidental discovery of the sickness

All six participants in the study experienced the unplanned, accidental discovery of a breast lump, signalling the sickness of which they were still not aware. Rather than the lump being diagnosed during medical check-ups or mammography screenings, the women themselves discovered the lump, almost by accident. Once discovered, the lump could not be ignored, but knowing what to do was not easy. There was a need to talk to others, to seek their advice, and to be guided in the most appropriate action.

> *The baby played with my breast from time to time. It was painful, so I tried squeezing it. Milk oozed and then there was blood. At that time, my husband was away from home and I didn't know who or where to turn to. I wrestled with the problem for some time and then went to a gynaecologist. I felt that I shouldn't take medicine. My neighbour told me that because pus had come out that I should go to the hospital, so I went to a large hospital.*

Husbands, neighbours, friends and physicians at various clinics and hospitals were consulted in order to have the significance of the lump explained and to be told what needed to be done. Often there were delays caused by inappropriate assessments and diagnoses. Most of the women themselves suspected that the lump was cancerous but relied on others to tell them what was wrong and what needed to be done, as in the following example:

> *At first, I felt a lump in my breast so I went to a private clinic. Since it was chest that was the problem, I thought I went to the right place. They took a chest X-ray and told me that it was just a little lump and*

that I should apply a warm towel at home. So I did that for a week. However, since it was not better I went to see a friend who had breast cancer. When I went to see her, I saw her breasts and they were like flowers in full bloom, strange in colour, yet beautiful. I didn't know that cancer would look like that. I asked her why it looked as it did and she told me that her brother had applied some sort of a pill to the growth. Then they did a moxacautery [the traditional practice of burning the dried leaves of the moxa plant on the skin as a counter-irritant] which turned it into such a red colour. On some days, it looked like a rabbit's tail and other days, it seemed as if it were not there. My husband urged me to go to the hospital. The doctor told me it was just a little residue and I went home very much relieved. However, it grew bigger after a month and this time the hospital said that it was cancer.

Searching for the cause

Once they were given the diagnosis of breast cancer, the women experienced the need to find the reason why the cancer had appeared and why it had happened to them rather than to someone else. They listed a number of possible internal and external causes and tried to review their lives and actions in order to identify which ones applied to them personally. As one of the women explained:

I was suddenly reminded of my bad character in relation to my breast cancer. I took more X-rays than anybody. I had several abortions. I ate a lot of meat. I have a very impatient character. All these things are very bad for my health.

The women were particularly reflective about their attributes as individuals, and the way they related with others and were treated by others. The sickness was seen as somehow related to a flaw in their character, with either an overly sensitive or an overly strong personality being seen as a likely cause of the cancer:

I think more sensitive people get it. When you are living with somebody, you have to be very patient about a lot of things, though I think that being patient is not the answer. You have to let go at times but the problem is that stress gets built up instead of being released. One of the very important ways to avoid sickness is to let go from time to time, and before I was able to do this. I used to get angry at my husband almost every day. Even little things made me angry. I wasn't able to control my anger. I think this led me to become very sensitive.

Other women were inclined to see cancer as having a more external cause, relationships with others being of particular importance. Listening to the women describe their lives, I sensed a deep unhappiness stemming from shattered dreams and feelings of helplessness; of being caught up in situations where others act and the women are left to cope with the effects:

> *The in-laws were nothing like what I had hoped they would be. They caused me a lot of physical and mental stress. What's more, my husband drinks a lot. He usually comes home very late, around midnight. Also, I am an introvert by nature so I didn't talk about my problems even when I went home [to my parents]. I didn't eat a lot of meat before I was married. I usually ate deon jang kook [traditional bean paste soup] or vegetables. I don't know whether it is hereditary or not but just thinking about it gives me a lot of stress. My husband is a very easygoing person and gets on well with other people. I, however, like to do things that I like and I don't like to do things that I don't like. So I think I get a lot of stress trying to get along with my husband.*

> *I think my husband was lonely at that time. He had an affair. I knew about it a year later. I had trusted him and had never imagined that he could do something like that. The conflicting emotions from that had great impact. Our baby wasn't living with us at that time and then suddenly my mother brought the baby back. The baby added to the stress. He was about 22 months old and I should have hugged my baby and looked after him but I wasn't able to do that. It was painful now that I think about it.*

> *I was physically and mentally stressed out while taking care of my mother-in-law for two years at home, and I lost a lot of weight because I was having such a hard time. I guess there was a lot of stress accumulated during the two years that I was there.*

Perhaps the most difficult to understand and come to terms with was the deep sense of wrongdoing that some of the women had—the idea that their cancer developed as a form of punishment. There was a perception that cancer does not happen to 'good' people. However good they had thought themselves to be, the appearance of cancer revealed that they had done something to deserve the punishment. In a strange way, linking cancer with 'being bad' or 'doing something wrong' was also reassuring, as evident from the following interview excerpts. If the cancer was the result of individual transgression then others were safe from it, and that seemed to provide some relief in a difficult situation. Yet, to the impact of the cancer and its treatment was added the heavy burden of moral responsibility which others did not share:

> *I don't think I could ever be gentle or good. My mind is really good but it is possible that underneath the good, there may be evil. It is possible to have bad thoughts while being good, which makes it impossible to be completely good as the books tell you to be. We lie and do bad things yet say that we don't do bad things. I am grateful though that there are people who are better than me who don't get the disease.*

> *Sometimes I think that I wasn't the only one who was bad in the past, so why me? Then I tell myself that it is because I was bad; so I am the one who deserves to get punished. My family members had nothing to do with it. I also think that it is because I did bad things that God is punishing me. I am the one who is responsible for dealing with the illness because I did the wrong things. I have a reasonably strong faith and it has helped me to believe in fairness. I deserve to get punished, so I will gladly receive the punishment.*

Fear of separation from family and present life

Whatever the suspected cause of cancer, its diagnosis brought with it anxiety and fear. It was almost as though the diagnosis was a death sentence and there was a sense of inevitability that death would come sometime soon. Yet in the midst of this personal crisis, the women talked not of a personal fear of death but of fear and concern for their children. Once again, their own concerns and aspirations were given second place as their thoughts turned to the future and their children's needs for motherly love and care. They envisaged a future in which they would no longer be present to take care of their families. They could see that the adults would readjust to their absence (and perhaps were doing so already), but they were concerned for their children and how the loss of their mother would affect them.

> *I think about my children the most. I pity them the most. I have lived as long as I can but the children are still growing . . . they need me. If I am not there their grandmother [would look after them], or their father can get married again, but the children, I pity them the most.*

> *I thought when my husband came home late it was very insensitive of him. Then I came home from the hospital and he told me that he didn't really feel like coming home because he felt restless. We do not really tell each other about the pain we are feeling. He drives a truck so he*

> *comes home once every two or three days. He never complains about being in pain. Stomach-aches or headaches are not even considered painful enough to mention. After hearing the diagnosis I was worried about the children. I couldn't sleep because I was worrying about them.*

Loss of one's habitual being after mastectomy

The surgery and the loss of a breast resulted in a visible change to the body which some of the women found difficult to accept. Some avoided, and were encouraged to avoid, looking at the scar and seeing their changed appearance. Their bodies were marred and no longer presentable to others, particularly their husbands. Once again personal difficulties, the courage needed to face their altered image in the mirror and to come to terms with the changes, were made secondary to the need to consider others and how others might react to their disfigured, imperfect bodies:

> *I feel guilty towards my husband, about having only one breast. Going out to meet my friends makes me feel uncomfortable. I don't feel like going anywhere.*

> *I felt that I could never go to the public baths again. My biggest worry was going to the public baths. I now bathe at home.*

> *I feel very awkward when others say something. I feel a little sore and I feel as if I have lost a part of my body forever. I looked at my wound [for the first time] after 15 days.*

> *I thought it would be my own personal problem as it will not show outwardly, but the sadness I felt after the operation was overwhelming. When I was being injected [with chemotherapy], my hands were like the leftover burnt twigs.*

In spite of such challenges to one's embodied being, the impact of the surgery was less devastating than the impact of chemotherapy which followed. It was not only that the bodily changes became more visible, but that the experience for these women became a nightmare. It was as if their body and soul were separated; they felt ill and distressed, as if they were living in a strange body intent on distressing them further. Their lack of control over their own bodies and what was being done to them made the weeks and months even more difficult to bear:

I lost a lot of hair. After being injected twice, the loss of hair became greater. It felt creepy to see hair as long as mine dropping off. I looked at my body and felt very melancholy.

I shook all over from the injections [of chemotherapy]. I had no energy. For six months, I begged them to reduce the amount of medication. The doctor told me that I could take the medication instead of radiation therapy because I was still young. But when I took the medicine, I became very restless, going all over the town; unable to eat, vomiting, lying down, sitting down, being restless, being injected, screaming. Whenever I feel mentally distressed I feel like screaming at the top of my voice.

What medical texts describe as the side effects of drugs used in chemotherapy, the women experienced as powerful forces controlling their bodies and threatening their very survival. Their familiar, habitual bodies no longer existed for them. Instead, they were driven by unknown forces and made to lead impossible lives. They felt profoundly anxious and uncomfortable, unable to sleep or rest, unable to find relief:

I am anxious to the point of terror. I feel anxious and I shake all over. So I try to sleep. I feel a lot better after I sleep. It's so hard when I can't sleep after receiving medication. When I received it for the first time without getting any sleep, I was shaking all over and it felt like it was taking about 100 hours for the medication [to be infused]. People who haven't gone through it will never understand. It's like a mouse who is terrified in front of a cat, or it's like facing an electric chair, physically and mentally; like on TV.

I had no problems when I was being treated with radiation therapy but when it came to the chemotherapy, I felt like dying. I received it for a year and they said that I could go crazy without actually being sick anywhere. It is like that. I feel restless, I can't sleep even when I take sleeping pills. I take the medication without sleeping a wink. Then I feel nauseated. That is the most difficult period.

What the women so poignantly described was the anguish and the nightmare that the months of chemotherapy became for them. It was as though their bodies were not only constantly assaulted but being pushed to the brink of disintegration. Even when the chemotherapy was concluded the nightmares did not always stop.

They say that it [chemotherapy] destroys all parts of the body. Let's suppose that a fly sat on a sheet of glass. Then to catch the fly, I hit

> *it with a hammer. The fly dies but the glass is shattered into pieces. So the cells in my body are not reduced but the whole body suffers from being shattered. All the bodily functions get destroyed. The pain was so intense during the [chemotherapy] treatment.*

> *I received it five times and I felt mentally ill. I thought I should lie in bed but it didn't help. I felt as if I was floating in the air; my body separated from my soul; my body twisted all over. It felt to me like the people I see in videos where they shake all over before electric torture. It's just like that. For a while I was afraid of the nights because of the torture. Even when I don't get injected I feel as if I have been injected on some nights.*

Drawing on others' support

In living through the experience of mastectomy and chemotherapy, the women in the study reported feeling largely alone. They carried the burden of personal responsibility for the sickness, struggled through the nightmare of chemotherapy, and worried what would happen to their children when they were no longer there to care for them. Yet for some there was external support; they felt encouraged and safe when able to rely on others. Husbands and mothers were seen as the principal sources of family support, even though in some cases the husbands were unable or unwilling to provide such support. When available, the presence of husbands or mothers was reassuring and comforting:

> *I received a lot of support from my husband. The best thing is to have your spouse being there beside you to support you. In some cases, women like having their mothers beside them. You feel secure when they are there and insecure if they are not there.*

Female friends and colleagues were also supportive, often in very practical ways, bringing special food and providing the financial assistance that is traditionally given in times of need:

> *Some colleagues brought ox-tail soup and some colleagues left money in envelopes when they came. When money from all the envelopes was added up later it was enough to pay for the cost of hospital treatment for a year.*

Some of the study participants talked of helpful information they obtained from books, while others stressed the need to rely on their doctors as the ones who knew best. In this context, nurses were not seen as sources of much-needed information about post-operative care, or about chemotherapy and how to cope with its effects. Nor were they seen as sources of personal support. Nurses did not offer information, even though the women felt strongly that they needed to know more about what was happening to them. The women, on the other hand, did not initiate conversations nor tell nurses how they felt or what they wanted to know.

Changing attitudes to life and its priorities

It would be difficult to live through the experience of cancer and possible death without stopping to think about life and its meaning. For some of the women in the study personal reflection resulted in a simple re-evaluation of how they should act and what they valued most. They stopped to listen, to be quiet, to meditate. They did not feel the urge to make instant decisions. Such changes, although simple, had quite profound effects. It was as if the women wanted life to slow down so that they could savour and appreciate each moment:

> *I was very outgoing but now I have changed. I was very much an extrovert but now I don't speak as much, nor do I laugh as much. My mind is more peaceful. Before, when I became angry I let it out immediately, but now I don't do that any more. I just feel at peace. Yes, I have become more peaceful. I think about things twice before I rush into doing something.*

> *I realise that I don't need people or money after all. The rich people may like it but for those who are fighting for their life, their health is the best blessing of all. The next important thing is to have three meals a day and it is the best blessing.*

For the majority of the women the struggle to come to terms with their experience and to find meaning in it was deeply spiritual. In some cases the spiritual quest for consolation and understanding took the women deeper into their cultural roots, in others towards some form of Christian understanding of God. Sometimes there was a blending of spiritual traditions in a very personal journey towards greater self-understanding and acceptance. What the women in the study had in common was the commitment of time and effort to this spiritual quest—time and effort for prayer, for reflection, for creative expression. Often it was a very disciplined, focused time, where they created their own space and sense of being. The deep thoughtfulness and some of the pain of reflecting on one's life and its purposes is best captured in the words of the women themselves:

After the mastectomy my hair began to drop off. I started to paint pictures which show a praying scene with lotus leaves floating on water which showed my state of mind. When I did that, I felt light and peaceful. This pain is not mine alone. About three hundred people came and encouraged me to get well and I thought, 'How can I lose courage?' I thought that the only thing that I can do to repay their kindness is to get well, and so it was possible to paint such a picture. Sometimes when I don't paint and can't sleep I lock my door and I recite a prayer, or I bow several times to make some kind of religious act.

I intend to go to church. At first I wasn't interested in church at all. Now, whenever I pray to God I feel my fears diminishing. I also think that there are people who are worse off than me and that I am lucky that it is not worse. I feel like clinging to God because when I die, I will finally go to him. So I want to cling to him.

I relied on God mentally a lot. I was afraid and scared so I wanted someone to rely on. I begged him that I was repentant about the bad things that I had done, so wouldn't he please let me live. I believe that God is eternal and omnipotent, so he has enough power to take care of me. I sometimes get tired of him and sometimes not. But now he is a big help to me. I try my best to reform my bad points and obey him. His words are so full of wonder and I try hard. I think we live through our lives committing sins. I thank him with all my heart inside. I thank him for letting the things happen to me as they did. I did not believe in him then but I pleaded with him to let me off just this once, and I will do better next time if he will just give me one more chance. So I began to pray every morning at dawn.

Writing gave me a chance to look back on my life. I cried a lot, but it wasn't because I was resentful or because someone had been mean to me. I was crying against truth. I will accept it gracefully and try to do my best. So while I was feeling like this, I made a sculpture with petals. I felt that as the petals came together one by one, anything was possible. I was nothing in this big universe and we all live alone, but I realised that I was someone valuable. That value extended to others, which made me realise about the pain others are going through as well. This made me more confident and important. I finished this reflection with praying, checking for any pride in my mind. It is a joyful thing that I have done the things that I have done in this world and that I am now learning to discipline myself. I look into my clear mind and sometimes feel pain, sometimes joy . . . Sometimes I feel ashamed and in pain but I think that it lasts just for a moment. I will be good and pure. While I tell myself that, I feel myself being purified. This sensation continues and when painting a picture I don't think about whether I like it or not, but there is the act of bowing in front of it with singing and dancing of my own. There is purification here again. When I am alone this makes my mind gentle and soft, but when I am outside sometimes my words become rough. When this happens I feel very sorry. I hope I can do this, but it is difficult. I pray that I will be able to do it. This won't be possible without leading a religious life.

Rediscovering the importance of personal health

The reassessment of life and its priorities was also reflected in how the women used food, what exercise they engaged in, and how they reconciled sometimes contradictory advice from traditional herbal lore and Western medicine. While accepting advice from both sources, they also took time and care to do what they thought would be best for their health. They also showed great interest in any tests that would show whether they were acting appropriately:

The reason I ate a lot of meat is that when I was getting the chemotherapy, the doctor told me that I will have shortage of blood, so to eat accordingly. I did, but I ate only lean meat, without any fat. I was eating this when other people told me not to eat meat, and I was worried that I would have a relapse. The meat would have a lot of preservatives in it. After my illness, I never put seasoning in the food. I use anchovies to cook soup. I don't eat meat anymore. My blood and iron are all at a normal level.

Most of the women seemed to favour traditional vegetarian dishes and fish or other seafood over red meat, fried food and food served in fast-food restaurants. Particular herbs, thought to have beneficial properties, would be added to such a diet:

I only eat vegetables now. I buy parsley and boil it to eat. I heard that parsley filters your blood and because my blood was clouded up, I ate raw pine leaves and parsley and I bought burdocks to eat. I eat any sort of vegetable. With rice, I put in burdocks, anchovies, a little sesame oil and fish, instead of meat.

Some resisted using Western medical remedies such as aspirin for minor ailments, preferring to rely on traditional herbal preparations; other women were less confident in dealing with even minor health problems. Whatever the approach, there was a common thread of carefulness about one's health—attentiveness to early symptoms and concern about doing that which would be most beneficial, whether drawing on Western or traditional Korean remedies:

> *I didn't take medicine even when I had a cold. I boiled the ginseng and Korean quince and raw radish with the skin still on it. I've heard that there is high water content in the radish skin. I eat all sorts of mountain vegetables and after doing aerobic exercises I take a shower, and it feels good.*

> *Nowadays, I go to the hospital once I feel that I am on the verge of getting a cold. Before, I tried to fix everything at home. Before the operation, I sweated a lot and nowadays I quickly go to the hospital as soon as I see any symptoms, or I take a sauna at home. I try everything that is not too harmful by taking Western medicine as well as Korean herb medicine.*

Recognising that one is ultimately alone

The experience of developing breast cancer and undergoing a mastectomy involved a great deal of anxiety, fear and stress for the women who took part in this study. They reported a need for support from others and for the help that their family and friends provided during this time. Yet, ultimately, they felt that much of what they were experiencing could not be shared with others. This was particularly so for the women who lacked their husbands' support. Their need to confide their innermost fears and to be reassured and comforted went unmet:

> *My husband doesn't even ask me how I am. When I tell him that I hurt somewhere he asks [how I feel] just for the sake of it. I have to bear it all alone. Where can I go and talk about this?*

> *I was fearful of the pain. I shook all over every night after I had chemotherapy. The fear was inside me. When I tried to tell this to my husband he would get angry, so I would force myself to control it. The important thing is to win the fight within myself.*

The realisation that the struggle was something happening within them, something that others could not fully comprehend, made the women feel that ultimately they were alone. If they were to win the fight, it would be by conquering their inner fears, something others could not do for them:

There is a book called The Pilgrim's Progress. *In the book, facets of human character are depicted in vivid detail. In order to get to heaven, the pilgrim starts off on a journey and during the journey he goes through a lot of difficulties. In one scene, he crosses bridges that are terrifying. But if I were to look at it more closely, the fear is inside and not outside.*

Learning to live in the shadow of death

However hard the women tried to deal with their fears and sense of aloneness, and however hard they tried to develop an attitude of acceptance, quietness and serenity, thoughts of death were never too far away. Their faith was fragile and their confidence easily shaken. Even minor symptoms appeared as omens of recurrence of cancer and death.

I think about death and there is always the fear of a relapse. I mean if I hurt only a little I immediately think that it must be a relapse and I get fearful. I do not have complete assurance that I will get well.

Once made acutely aware of their own mortality, the women became more aware of death happening to others around them. Even television dramas acted as strong reminders of death—not as something fictional, but as real and very close:

After I had surgery, I thought about death and I thought that it was my destiny. I felt afraid, but if there is no relapse [I thought that] I would live forever. I think only about death now and I know I won't die right after the operation, but then I think again and I think that I will die later, or that I will die when there is a relapse. I know death is around me. In [the TV drama] Love and Separation, *I feel a lot of empathy with the heroine Sun-Ju. Fear, depression. Why is the title 'separation'? I worry a lot that the heroine might die.*

CONCLUSION

For Korean women middle age is expected to be a time of growing maturity and of focusing on virtuous living—cultivating the mind rather than paying attention to physical appearance. The cultural expectation is that by this stage of life women will have learned to dedicate their time and energies to caring and tending to the needs of others. Rather than focusing on their own needs and desire for personal fulfilment, they often live in a way which gives primacy to their husbands, children, parents-in-law and community.

The sudden and often frightening appearance of breast cancer served to turn the attention of the women in this study to themselves. Not used to placing themselves first or acting independently of family and friends, the women experienced diagnostic procedures, mastectomy and subsequent chemotherapy as a time of great stress and turbulence. This applied not only to the bodily discomfort, pain and distress they experienced over many months, but also to the need to find meaning in what was happening to them and a renewed sense of purpose in a life which had become profoundly different.

Perhaps the most distressing experience for the women was the process of searching for the cause of breast cancer and the eventual attribution to something within their inner or outward being—inappropriate diet, a sensitive or forceful nature, stressful family relationships or bad deeds. They saw it as something for which they were personally responsible. Added to this burden of (complete or partial) personal responsibility for the development of breast cancer, was the realisation of their ultimate existential aloneness. However supportive others tried to be, the pain, the uncertainty and the innermost fears were theirs alone. These women wanted others' closeness and support, but were afraid of how others would react to the malignant nature of their disease, the hard scar where a soft breast had once been, and the effects of chemotherapy.

Western medicine offered the women in this study a reprieve from cancer, a mastectomy to remove the tumour, and chemotherapy to try to destroy any remaining traces. However the treatment was destructive of much more than cancer—the treatment as much as the cancer had shattered their bodies and their lives. In their search for a renewed sense of health and wholeness, the women resorted to a life of careful attentiveness. They were careful about the food they ate, the traditional herbs and remedies they took, and the minor symptoms that appeared from time to time. To win over their inner fears and to find the courage to face the future the women engaged in a spiritual quest, often involving creative activities. It was in the process of painting, sculpting, writing, meditating and praying that they started to gain a sense of their own importance as individual persons and their place in the universe—not so much as wives, daughters or mothers, but as persons in their own right. From a somewhat marginalised place occupied by middle-aged women in Korea, they felt that they were able to move centre stage. While they continued to feel that they lived in the shadow of death, never confident that the cancer would not recur, there was a kind of strength that came from conquering their fears and a serenity achieved through spiritual reflection and the reordering of priorities.

It is something of an indictment on the nurses who cared for these women during their hospitalisation and subsequent chemotherapy treatment that they seem to have made so little impact on the women's experiences. They needed information about breast cancer, assistance to explore treatment alternatives available to them, support to come to terms with their changed bodies, guidance and encouragement in sharing their experience with family and friends, and information and support during the months of the 'nightmare' of chemotherapy. Phenomenological research can assist Korean nurses to give more sensitive and appropriate care by providing descriptions of their patients' lived experiences and highlighting areas in which nurses can make a positive difference.

REFERENCES

Ali, N.S. & Khalie, H.Z. 1991 'Identification of stressors, level of stress, coping strategies, and coping effectiveness among Egyptian mastectomy patients' *Cancer Nursing* vol. 14, no. 5, pp. 232–9

Cancer Registration Office, National Medical Centre 1994 *Cancer Report* Ministry of Health, Seoul

Cho, Y.J. 1991 *Body and Art* Art Education Co., Seoul

Choe, D.S. 1992 'A study of the relationship between social support networks and self-esteem in middle-aged women' unpublished dissertation, Ewha Womans University, Seoul

Chung, B.J. 1988 *A Theory of Personality and Identity of Korean Middle-aged Women* I-Mun Press, Seoul

Chung, B.R. 1991 'The process of adjustment in women with breast cancer: an emotional experience' unpublished dissertation, Yonsei University, Seoul

Da Jong Kyung 1995 *The Canonical Textbook of Won Buddhism* Won Kwang Co., Iri, Korea

Dong Eu Bo Gam 1610/1992 revised by Hong Moon Wha, Deung Ti Co., Seoul

Han, K.S. 1991 'The process of adjustment in women with breast cancer' unpublished dissertation, Yonsei University, Seoul

Harris, J.R., Hellman, S., Henderson, I.C. & Kinne, D.W. 1991 *Patient Rehabilitation and Support: Breast Disease* Lippincott, Pa.

Kim, D-H. 1994 *Rain, Rain, Rain* Jayou-Munhak Press, Seoul

Kim, J.E. 1983 *Human Development Process* Jeon Mang Sa Press, Seoul

Kim, M.J. 1989 'A study of factors associated with middle age crisis' unpublished dissertation, Ewha Womans University, Seoul

Kim, T.Y. 1993 *The Engineering Professor's Poem* Adtec Press, Seoul

Lee, W.H. 1992 'The conflict and the coping patterns of Korean middle-aged women' *Journal of Adult Nursing* vol. 4, no. 2, pp. 136–46

Lindberg, A.M. 1959 *The Gift from the Sea* (Korean trans. I. Lee 1992) The World of Language Press, Seoul

Northouse, L.L. 1989 'The impact of breast cancer on patients and their husbands' *Cancer Nursing* vol. 12, no. 5, pp. 276–84

Oh, S.M. 1993 'Women's breast' *Dong Ah* (Daily News), Seoul, 7 June, p. 32

Park, H.K. (1986) 'A study of factors related to depression in mastectomy patients following discharge from hospital' unpublished dissertation, Pusan University, Pusan, Korea

Shin, S.K. & Park, H.I. 1993 'Stress and coping strategies experienced by middle-aged married women' *Kaemyung University Science Research Report* vol. 19, pp. 16–24

van Manen, M. 1990 *Researching Lived Experience* State University of New York Press, New York

Wong, C.A. & Bramwell, L. 1992 'Uncertainty and anxiety after mastectomy for breast cancer' *Cancer Nursing* vol. 15, no. 5, pp. 363–71

Yeo Sung Dong Ah 1995 'Animals and dreams' *Dong Ah*, Seoul, March, p. 323

Yeun, D.B. 1993 'Perception of the AIDS epidemic by women in their 50s' *Cho-Sun* (Daily News), 2 July, p. 18

six

On living with schizophrenia

JO ANN WALTON

This chapter is drawn from the author's PhD study, which examined what it is like to live with a schizophrenic illness. Ten adults who had been diagnosed with schizophrenia, each living in the community and taking regular medication, were visited and interviewed several times over a period of sixteen months. They were asked about their experiences, their illness and its effects on their everyday lives. The participants, who were contacted through an intermediary after ethical approval for the study was gained, included seven men and three women. They ranged in age from 21 to 64 years, and their occupations, paid or unpaid, included a painter, a writer, an academic and an educator for a voluntary organisation. Some participants were unemployed. All had been diagnosed with schizophrenia at least two years prior to the study; in fact one had been living with the illness for over 40 years. Most participants were living in their own homes, although four were in supported or supervised accommodation.

In this chapter, nine of the ten study participants are represented. The other participant features in different aspects of the original work (Walton 1995).

All names used in the chapter are fictional, although during the course of the research several participants requested that their real names be used. Although this request has not been met, acknowledgement is made to each of the study participants who gave so generously of their time and who shared their experiences so frankly and with such good humour. Without their help the study would never have been completed.

FEW ILLNESSES IN today's world are as baffling as schizophrenia. It is an enigma not only for those whose thoughts, perceptions, emotions and behaviour it so seriously disturbs, at least in its acute phases, but also for the generations of researchers, theoreticians and clinicians who have studied it since it was recognised as a distinct illness a hundred years ago. As one of the most serious of mental disorders, schizophrenia has been both researched extensively and feared widely.

The Latin saying 'Whom God wishes to destroy He first makes mad' is not far removed from the suggestion that schizophrenia is 'a sentence as well as a diagnosis' (Hall et al. 1985, cited in Torrey 1988, p. 1). The sense of tragedy conveyed in both these sayings is understandable. Schizophrenia is an illness whose cause (or causes) is unknown and for which there is no known prevention. Moreover, even though drug therapies are becoming increasingly successful in the control of symptoms and early intervention is holding promise for good prognosis in the young, there is no cure for schizophrenia. Estimates of recovery rates vary considerably, but it is widely held to be a long-term illness in the majority of cases. It has even been suggested that schizophrenia affects people so cruelly that it 'leads to a twilight existence, a twentieth-century underground man' (Torrey 1988, p. xv).

Little is known about what it is like to live with the illness—until quite recently the scientific community has paid only sporadic attention to the experience of schizophrenic patients. So, while there is a vast amount of literature on such aspects as brain pathology, neuropsychology and the clinical and neurological aspects of schizophrenia, we have limited knowledge about the experiences of people with the illness, or the effects the illness has on their lives.

In recent years prevailing humanitarian and economic rationales have resulted in a virtually universal move towards the closure of institutions for the mentally ill and the reintegration of those with mental illness into community settings. Many people who are diagnosed with a major mental illness may now never be hospitalised, or may receive hospital treatment for only a very brief time. As a consequence, people with mental illnesses are becoming more visible in the community, and some groups are becoming more effective in advocating on their own behalf.

The deinstitutionalisation movement and its attendant notion of community care have emphasised the need to take notice of differences in individual needs and people's quality of life (Bachrach 1988), while the need to learn more about the ways in which people with schizophrenia learn to cope with their symptoms has been identified as an important area for research (WHO 1991). Some excellent examples of work in this area can be found in such works as Barham and Hayward 1991, Goldschalx 1989, Leary et al. 1991 and Vellenga and Christenson 1994.

Of particular importance to nursing is the understanding of the *experience* of illness, defined by Kleinman (1988, p. 3) as 'the innately human experience of symptoms and suffering', rather than disease itself, which is equated with pathology. Morse and Johnson (1991) assert that understanding illness will lead to more effective healthcare. Indeed nurse researchers are becoming increasingly interested in the experience of living with persistent illness but, as yet, the knowledge base stemming from such interest is not sufficiently developed to guide nursing practice (Packard et al. 1991).

Aldiss (1989, p. viii) quotes Carl Jung as saying: 'All we see of the mentally ill regarding them from the outside, is their tragic destruction, rarely the life of that side of the psyche which is turned away from us.' The study on which this chapter is based was designed to try to see something of the side which is turned away.

A VERY BRIEF INTRODUCTION TO HEIDEGGER

In the thesis from which this chapter is drawn (Walton 1995), considerable use is made of the ideas and work of the German phenomenologist Martin Heidegger, particularly his early work in *Being and Time* (1927/1962). In this chapter I have endeavoured to minimise references to Heidegger in order to retain a more readable style. Much of Heidegger's work is not easy to grasp, and I wish neither to baffle readers nor to use up space explaining complex ideas. However, there are a few of Heidegger's concepts that are especially relevant to the points I wish to make here, and I trust that readers will bear with me in the few references to his work that are necessary in order that these points are made clear.

Heidegger's writing concentrated on the nature of human existence in its 'everydayness'. It is, he said, through our everyday dealings with things in the world and with other people, in our goals and projects, the intentions we hold, and the way we live out our hopes and values, that we are defined.

Heidegger used the word *Dasein* to refer to human existence itself (literally translated, *Dasein* means 'being there'). *Dasein*, he says, is *thrown* into existence. The notion of *thrownness* relates to the fact that we are already in the world, and that we are there *as we are*, in a world which 'was not of our making but with which we are nonetheless stuck' (Hall 1993, p. 137). In the world we are *thrown* into situations with certain possibilities and limitations. In Heidegger's view, we are not simply in the world as entities among a world of other entities, we are not things among other things (Stewart & Mikunas 1974). Rather, *Dasein*, self and world are one (Dostal 1993, p. 155):

> Dasein . . . is defined as being-in-the-world. The hyphens, almost as awkward in German as they are in English, are indicative of the fact that, as Dasein, self and world are a unity. The world is not something external but is constitutive of Dasein. We are born into a world whose culture and history make us what we are. The Christian view that 'we are in the world, but not of the world' is transformed. We are both in and of the world. 'Worldliness' is an ontological property of Dasein; it is our context of involvements.

Heidegger's view is not a fatalistic and deterministic one. Rather it suggests that each of us is an individual, who must come up against history and the future in such a way that we make our own life according to our choices, within certain limits that constrain us. We are shaped by cultural and historical understandings, but have a certain, situated freedom within which to choose what we make of our lives. Since our world includes our history and our cultural orientations, the understandings that society has and has had about mental illness colour the beliefs held by sufferers, families and professional carers.

In this chapter I will concentrate on the way in which illness and treatment impacted on the study participants' experience of Being-in-the-world. Other aspects of Being-in-the-world include relationships with others, managing life with an ongoing illness, and the whole process of making choices in life, depending on the things that matter to each individual. While some of these aspects of Being-in-the-world will be mentioned in this chapter, it is not possible to do justice to all of them here. Readers who are interested in following the discussion further are referred to the original study (Walton 1995) for more detail.

REALISING THAT ONE IS UNWELL

It is not a simple matter to acquire a diagnosis of schizophrenic illness. The early signs of schizophrenia can be insidious and may be more easily recognised in retrospect. Commonly health professionals do not name the illness until months after the onset of symptoms, and people who are becoming ill, and sometimes those around them, may find it difficult to believe that anything is seriously wrong.

As Liz explained, in the normal course of life, people doubt neither the evidence of their senses nor their own beliefs. When she was acutely ill, Liz believed that she was clairvoyant and that she had discovered some connection between the Russians and the weather. In spite of what sound to outsiders like most unusual thoughts, Liz carried on with her life as she always had:

> *It felt pretty normal actually. Although it was . . . it wasn't normal at all. But . . . when I had no insight . . . you don't doubt yourself, you know, you don't sort of think oh, you know . . . well you don't have any doubts about, well I try not to anyway. You make a decision and you think . . . or you think about something and you come up with the answer and you don't . . . you don't think oh, you know, I could be wrong, you know, and get all stressed out about it, you sort of stick to your decision and go about your business, you know. And that's what it's like, you know, you just make up your mind, I mean however bizarre it is, you know, and just go about doing something about it. So that's . . . feels pretty normal. Sounds strange, eh?*

Although in retrospect Liz recognised these thoughts as symptomatic of her psychotic illness, at the time she did not doubt her perceptions or the reasoning which explained them. Judith told her parents that she was hearing voices but they did not accept this. In contrast, Michael's friends were aware that something was wrong considerably earlier than he was:

> *Then the two chaps I was travelling around with in Europe they found that I was very slow. In my actions and speech and everything. And they always used to have me on about it. And I could never understand why they used to have me on about it all the time because as far as*

> *I was concerned I was keeping up with them. But they could see differently, you know, and that was one of the things that really stood out, you know, but at that stage I never realised there was anything wrong with me.*

Chris expressed concern at the way in which social welfare benefits may enable people who are seriously ill to 'disappear' in our society—away from the public eye—in circumstances that may be desperate. Keeping to oneself may be one way to avoid treatment which, as Chris explained, can be very frightening to contemplate:

> *When you have a system where you're bankrolled, but on the dole and stuff . . . like my illness wasn't diagnosed because I was able to stay on the dole for all those years and I was in hell, I was in a living hell. I was ill. But I could collect the dole and live in a private hotel, not speak to anyone, everyone was saying go to a hospital, go to hospital; I wasn't going to go to a hospital unless I was forced because I'd seen* One Flew Over The Cuckoo's Nest *and I'd seen it through certain eyes. And I just thought it was a nightmare. I just identified with Jack Nicholson. I saw it again after I'd been in hospital and I identified with the nurse. [Laughs] Nurse Rat Shit.*[1] *I could see it. I thought what a marvellous person she is.*

The symptoms of illness itself may also lead to a fear of treatment, as Judith described:

> *The first time I went to the hospital I was sure that I was being watched. So I thought people were watching me, things like that. And I said to [my partner] David, 'I'm not safe.' That's how it made you feel, like you weren't safe around anybody.*

As their illness developed, the normal way of Being-in-the-world for each of these people came under challenge. Liz had strange new powers of clairvoyance which required contemplation and action. Judith heard voices which disturbed her yet which her parents were dubious about, and she felt frightened everywhere she was, even when presenting for the help she later realised she needed. Michael was puzzled by the reaction of his friends who appeared, in his view, to be unfairly intolerant of his actions and manner. Chris was, in his words, 'in a living hell', yet his understanding of a popular film of the time left him in very real fear of seeking or being sent for treatment. While he later laughed at his interpretation, it was his experience at the time, a reflection of the world into which he had been thrown. Each of these people conveyed their certainty about their thoughts, behaviour and judgement in the face of experiences that sound unusual and, in some instances, very difficult for anyone else to believe. But at the time these people had no reason to doubt their own judgement.

RECONCEPTUALISING ONE'S BEING-IN-THE-WORLD

The recognition that they were unwell and required treatment, however slowly it dawned, led each of the participants to reconceptualise their Being-in-the-world. Previous explanations for perceptions, actions and the cause of unusual experiences had to be overturned.

Michael, Chris, Roger and Jack all believed that they had been sick from a very early age. Since this was the way they had always been, or so they believed, it was difficult for them to accept that they were unwell. Another reason for participants not thinking they were unwell was that there were other ways of explaining 'different' ideas, beliefs and behaviours. Chris succinctly described the role of changing fashion in ideas as contributing to his inability to acknowledge a problem:

> *I think of it as me being sick from the day I was born really.*
>
> (Do you know a lot of people have told me that. But you just didn't know till later?)
>
> *No . . . because there are all sorts of other things mixed up in it, there are current political ideas and fashions that fit in with your illness so you think that's . . . you grasp those and you don't think I'm being ill, you think I'm being fashionable [laughs].*

Things were a little different for Judith and Liz, who both acknowledged the regular and heavy use of street drugs such as marijuana and hash oil and felt that this had possibly been the precipitating cause of their illness. In addition, Judith was involved in studying the zodiac, tarot cards and other occult practices and was uncertain about dismissing the power of the spirit world in having something to do with her problems.

Whatever the cause of the illness, coming to terms with it *as an illness*, and reconceptualising one's Being-in-the-world in this light, was a gradual process with weighty consequences. Some of the problems that arose for participants stemmed from having to deal with the prejudices of others once their illness had been given a name. Other consequences arose from treatment, and its effects on the body as well as on the mind.

ILLNESS, TREATMENT AND BEING-IN-THE-WORLD

Both illness and treatment affect the whole of one's Being. Although schizophrenia is thought of as primarily a mental illness, in fact it has major effects on the body as it is lived, as do hospitalisation, drugs and other therapies such as ECT (electroconvulsive therapy). There is no way to separate, for instance, the sensation of hearing voices from the experience of hearing; nor is there a way to separate visual hallucinations from the experience of sight, or tiredness or fear from an experience of body, mind and spirit together. One *hears* voices, *sees* things, *feels* tired, anxious, restless or afraid. Each of these symptoms is an experience that affects Being-in-the-world as a whole.

Different symptoms bothered participants to varying degrees. No two participants had identical symptoms, although several were described in very similar ways. Since all the participants were taking medication it would be difficult to determine in any objective way which symptoms and experiences were related to illness and which to treatment, and to what degree. Although on the whole the participants were clear as to which was which, in a phenomenological study such as this the distinction is not critical: having the illness meant that all the participants took regular medication, so both the illness and its treatment had, at the time of the study, become part of their Being-in-the-world.

HALLUCINATING

Hallucinations, perceptions for which there are no external stimuli, are a common symptom in schizophrenic illness, and these were described in vivid detail by those participants who had experienced them. Hallucinations may involve any of the senses. In the following cases they were auditory, visual or tactile, but whatever the type, they had powerful effects on the person experiencing them. As they are lived, hallucinations are not simply mental or perceptual phenomena. They affect the whole of a person's Being-in-the-world.

Lucy suffered from frightening hallucinations when she was most unwell and, as she explained, she still occasionally experiences some of these sensations. She began by describing how real the voices sounded, her statement reinforcing Liz's earlier explanation of believing what she heard:

> *Because they're so normal sounding, well it's not normal . . . but because they're so clear and coherent you think well . . . sometimes*

> *you get embarrassed because you think, cor, everybody's listening to that. And why isn't anybody going red, you know, things like that. Sometimes they do it now and it's just a silly little kind of thing. Cos I probably get visions worse than voices now. But it's in a very obscure way like in trees and like I used to, when I used to walk to the dairy or just up the road, I'd have a thing about rats. I'd stand on rats, you know, things like that. And you can feel them squish between your toes. So then I'd never walk barefoot for years because I'd think, 'Shit, I'm going to stand on another bloody rat.' And I went to the dairy [corner shop] one day and the rats were in my long hair. And I said, 'I'm not going to that dairy.' So I looked in the mirror and they were all crawling and creeping and they had those long tails and they had like blood between their teeth and it was disgusting. And I thought if I go into that dairy she's going to think what am I doing putting bloody rats in my hair just to scare her or something. So I had to turn back halfway. And worms. I can't walk at night when it's been raining. I still can't do it now because I don't like killing animals. Snails. And eating stones, chewing on stones, when I'm eating my porridge or something. I can chew, chew, chew like I'm stepping on snails, but in my mouth. Some things have stayed behind.*

Jack does not hear voices but there are times when he experiences strange visual images:

> (What happens while you're hallucinating? What sort of things?)
>
> *Oh just jagged yellow lines, all queer and then me* [sic] *brain goes . . . part of me brain wants to go to sleep and part of it's frightened to go to sleep. It's horrible and I get horrible bizarre fantastic horrible pictures in me brain but I usually get to sleep sooner or later and then sleep it off.*

Jack sleeps off his unpleasant hallucinatory experiences whereas Lucy, in the past, has resorted to some extreme physical acts, including cutting off her long hair and picking large areas of skin from her hands, in an attempt to stop her hallucinations.

Whether pleasant or distressing, when the hallucinations cease they may be missed, as both Lucy and Liz explained. Liz noted that she had not realised that 'normal people' (a term she herself used) did not hear voices in the way she did. Lucy became quite depressed when her voices first left and admitted that, horrible as they had been, she felt lonely without them.

The hallucinatory experience, involving hearing, seeing or feeling, frequently interferes with other activities. As Lucy explained, it may also make the conduct of activities that are usually taken for granted very taxing, if not impossible:

> *And then a friend, he's an artist, he picked me up one morning when I didn't go to work and I was just walking the streets near where I live, he took me to his place. And I couldn't, I couldn't . . . I didn't know what he was saying. I could see his mouth move but I couldn't actually hear what he was saying because I was so . . . [the voices were] blabbing so loud. But I never hear voices inside my head. It's around me. And when I'm hearing eight at a time and somebody's trying to talk to me you can imagine how confusing that is. Because you're listening to that one, that one, that one, that one, that one, and then you've got to listen to the person who's actually in front of you.*

Hallucinations are a well-recognised symptom of schizophrenic illness. Other less well-known perceptual changes may precede or accompany a psychotic episode or occur at other times, as detailed in the following section.

FEELINGS OF UNFAMILIARITY AMONG THINGS IN THE WORLD

Several of the study participants reported episodes of feelings of unreality or strangeness. Jack attempted to describe to me what these feelings of unreality are like:

> *What else can I tell you? . . . Ask some questions about . . . about schizophrenia. Oh I get feelings of unreality occasionally. Not occasionally, rarely, but I do get them. Do you know what that means?*
>
> (Tell me what it means.)
>
> *Well it's different, that's only way I can sum it up. You know I might go . . . I had it the other day after he changed me* [sic] *pills. Dr Gerard . . . I went down to [hospital] and I had a different mental impression, in the . . . in me brain, to what I normally did. That was just walking in there. Things seemed, not actually different, yeah sort of different, I don't mean the furniture was different but . . . I felt differently about it. And you know you get feelings . . . unreality to what you normally get. Different to what you normally get.*
>
> (It looks different, or it . . .)
>
> *Well it doesn't look different, no . . .*

(It feels different?)

Well . . . I feel different about it. Yeah it seems . . . it seems sort of different to me, I have a different outlook about it, that sort of thing, you know. You get sort of feelings of unreality it . . . it can be . . . if it's strong it's disturbing and worrying. It worries you a bit. You feel unsure of yourself. That's the way to sum it up, you feel unsure of yourself. I have heard it referred to as unreality and irreality and that but ah . . . it's just different. That's one of the things.

(They're quite difficult to describe some of these symptoms, aren't they?)

Mmm. Well you've got to liken it to something that you'll understand. You see if you've never had a total nervous breakdown you really don't know what it's like. You just don't . . . I can't put it into words to liken it to anything that will mean anything to you, you see. But you've got nothing to . . . you've got no . . . see, ah . . . [demonstrates how cup sits on saucer] this is a cup because this is a saucer. You've got . . . if this was the only thing in the world well it wouldn't have the same meaning to you because it's got a saucer, cup and a saucer, you can compare. And if I explain to you, you've got to be able to compare it to something that you know, understand and . . . and if you've never been through it, it's difficult to do that.

Although these feelings were difficult for the participants to explain, they appear to correspond closely to the notion of unreality which precedes an acute psychotic episode as described by Sass (1992). These feelings of unreality also closely fit the concept of *uncanniness* described by Heidegger (1927/1962), and can be analysed in terms of his notions of the breakdown of the *ready-to-hand. Uncanniness* may also be conceived of as *not-being-at-home*. In a state of anxiety one feels uncanny. It is a state in which 'everyday familiarity collapses' (Heidegger 1927/1962, p. 233). Anxiety in Heidegger's definition is a more complex state of mind than that which we take it to be in common usage. He suggests that we become anxious not about this thing or that thing, but rather in the face of Being-in-the-world as such. Things, particularly objects which may be used towards some end, are *ready-to-hand* when they are employed smoothly in practical activity. In those moments when we realise just how things are in the world, as separate from us, when there is nothing ready-to-hand, then we are anxious. In the quote above Jack describes, with some difficulty, how things became different *to* him. Their common, smooth functioning broke down and he was left puzzled and uncertain, unsure of *himself* in his relation to the things around him.

Jack remembered another, similar, experience involving his relation to things and people. The difficulty he had in finding words at the beginning of his description shows what a disturbing and strange experience this was for him:

> *So I've been in the state of total mental dep . . . intellectual . . . when people . . . Well just before I came out of [hospital] they had me delivering the mail. And I didn't know what I was doing. I know the letters went all . . . I probably lost half of them. I remember . . . I do remember a few words. I remember one of the girls there saying to one of the blokes that was in charge of the office, 'I don't think he knows what he's doing.' And he said, 'Let him persevere.' But some of the words they spoke there was no intellectual acknowledgement in me* [sic] *brain.*
>
> (The words didn't mean anything.)
>
> *Yeah me brain was intellectually numb.*

Experiences such as this are not easily articulated, and, for those who have not undergone them, are difficult to imagine. However, they clearly have an impact on the person whose perspective, relationships with the things about him and whole Being-in-the-world has been altered by such an experience.

Sass (1992, p. 45) writes of the perceptual and emotional experiences which accompany states such as that described by Jack above, suggesting that these experiences can give rise to 'the sense of radical alienness that some European psychiatrists have considered the best diagnostic indicator of schizophrenia'. Sass goes on to say (1992, pp. 45–6):

> To patients in this state of mind, the world is stripped of its usual meanings and sense of coherence and it therefore defies any standard description. Everything bristles with a new and overwhelming quality of definiteness and significance, yet patients cannot say what the special meanings they sense are, nor just what is important about the details that, in their ineffable specificity, so compel their attention. Even the most articulate schizophrenics are usually reduced to helplessly repeating the same, horribly inadequate phrase: everything is strange, or everything is somehow different.

A different kind of breakdown between body and world is described by Michael. He sometimes does maintenance work around his house but finds that his coordination is sometimes poor and that he occasionally has trouble with the tools he is using. This problem, which he conceptualised as one of poor coordination resulting from confused thinking, is another good demonstration of the unexpected unreadiness-to-hand of tools. In the ready-to-hand state, Michael's building proceeds smoothly, but at times he and the instruments are somehow 'out of sync' and the habitual smooth activity suddenly becomes derailed.

(You're practical?)

Oh yeah well being a carpenter you have to be. But I'm not very good on the tools though. I think my coordination is controlled by my thinking. That's getting back to this confusion bit where my mind gets confused, where I'm building something or . . . um . . . I get a bit confused and sidetracked and it means I'm not working my hands properly, controlling my tools properly. So things don't quite go right as . . . I never have been a very good carpenter actually. In theory it's all right, I can do the theory of it all right, but as far as handling the tools go, I'm not very good at times.

Michael's account contains a clear description of the breakdown of a smooth, non-reflective action. In such a state the body becomes aware of itself rather than simply being absorbed in practical activity. Indeed, Michael's consciousness of his difficulty with carpentry tools is very similar to Heidegger's classic description of the breakdown of the ready-to-hand, in which he uses the example of a hammer. As Heidegger describes it, things are ready-to-hand when we are engaged in smooth, everyday action such as hammering. When things are going smoothly we concentrate on the work rather than the tools, the latter being taken for granted as an extension of our actions in the world. When something goes wrong, however, and smooth functioning breaks down, we become aware of the hammer as a tool, separate from us. It suddenly becomes conspicuous and we see it as 'an equipmental Thing' (Heidegger 1927/1962, p. 103).

In Michael's case, it is not only the tools of which he becomes aware, but his own bodily functioning and his ability to coerce it into the smooth actions he plans and imagines. Participants in the study described not only the way in which they were aware of their bodily actions, but the way in which they might also become aware of their thoughts, which sometimes become overpowering and distracting.

BEING OCCUPIED WITH ONE'S THOUGHTS

Nearly all the study participants spoke of difficulties that arose for them in their everyday life as a result of a mind busy with thoughts. Sometimes this was simply a matter of having trouble concentrating—it was often possible to detect a participant's mind wandering off during interview sessions—and most participants said that they frequently experienced several thoughts at once. Many said that it was difficult to read for this reason. Interviews were quite tiring for several participants because of the effort they had to put in to concentrating. Most distressing were persistent, unhappy thoughts—confusion, worry, anxiety or fear—and these often took up considerable amounts of time for those who experienced them.

Chris reported lying in bed every night contemplating his life and whether he was yet ready for suicide. Judith spent a lot of time considering the nature of her illness and dwelling on ideas that there was some conspiracy involved. Roger said he felt 'anxiety towards life in general'. Michael talked of his confusion, emphasising the difficulty of his experiences, perhaps in order to make sure I did not minimise them:

> *Oh, not being able to think straight at times, um . . . like, um . . . trying to solve a problem, or um . . . solve a situation, and you get all confused, and you end up not knowing what to do and . . . but after a while you . . . after a period of time, suddenly realise what you should have done, and what you shouldn't have done, and . . . I suppose it happens to normal people though, doesn't it?*
>
> (Yeah, I'm sure.)
>
> *But in schizophrenic people, it's a lot worse, they get confused, and can't think straight.*

Even very simple, everyday tasks can become overshadowed by a mind which is busy with worrying thoughts, so that the work itself became an impossible task for Jack:

> *Well what I normally used to do, and love, worries me now, I don't do it. I try and do it . . . I've got to drive meself* [sic] *to do certain things at times. Force meself. For instance when I'm gardening I don't garden for an hour. I'll go out for ten minutes, come inside, have a cup of tea and a smoke . . . for ten minutes and then go out and do another ten minutes. I can't stick at it all day. I used to work . . . I worked for five years in the council and ah . . . I was there every day*

> *except when I went fishing, I took days off to go fishing. You know the whitebait season opened, I was away on opening day and things like that. I used to get time off. But I drove meself for five years until I became a leading hand in charge of the [job] and so . . . I could . . . I could do it then but I . . . as I say I get that way I can't even wash the dishes some nights.*

Worrying was something Jack claimed to be an expert at, suggesting to me that anything I could think of he could worry about. His returning to the house to smoke and drink tea was an occasion to let his thoughts roam and to do some worrying, as he explained it. The connection between thinking and physical inaction has parallels in other participants' descriptions of the effect of their illness on their body.

THE ALTERED BODY

Although schizophrenia is usually thought of as a *mental* illness, it incorporates a number of *physical* aspects. As it is lived, schizophrenia is experienced not just in terms of its cognitive manifestations, but bodily. While it is in some ways self-evident that human beings are bodily in the world, it is nonetheless sometimes easy for health professionals to overlook the physical ramifications of mental ill-health, or to minimise their significance when such problems are not connected to the primary symptoms of the illness. We know that it is the body that is treated with medications and that some of the more severe side effects of drugs are physical, yet we may forget the everyday implications of illness in terms of physical wellbeing and people's ability to undertake usual activities. The physical problems that arise as a result of illness and treatment are arguably more troubling for people, such as those in this study, who are ostensibly well, than are the perhaps more intense physical reactions which may be monitored during a period of acute illness and treatment. The 'well' must cope with physical symptoms that are ongoing and often quite disabling, yet there is little that health professionals can do to alleviate these symptoms, even when they are recognised.

The classification of the symptoms of schizophrenia into positive and negative as is found in textbook descriptions does not parallel the experience of people with the illness. For example, tiredness is not only experienced as a lack of energy, as something missing or absent; there are aspects of tiredness which are experienced as attributable to the *presence* of bodily sensations such as heavy limbs and slowed movement and thinking. There is another problem that arises in relation to the terms used to define the symptoms of schizophrenia. One of the commonly recognised 'negative' symptoms of schizophrenia is avolition/apathy (included in the majority of negative-symptom rating scales discussed by Schooler 1994). In New Zealand the term 'lack of motivation' is commonly used and it was spoken of by all study participants. The lived experience of the study participants was that this symptom belonged much more to the physical realm than to the psychological. Several participants in the study described lack of motivation as a feeling of tiredness or as difficulty in commencing or completing tasks, no matter how much they *wanted* to do them. If motivation is taken as a synonym of will, then the difficulty expressed is not really one of motivation but of propelling the body into the world.

In the previous extract Jack talked of needing to *force himself* to do things. He himself suggested that the problems he described were due to lack of motivation. Yet he is clearly not lacking in desire; rather he finds it difficult to have his body follow through with the actions he wishes to undertake.

For Michael 'lack of motivation' was a persistent problem, and the most troublesome symptom he had to deal with. He felt that he suffered from this problem to an unacceptable degree and that his difficulty in being able to do things because of tiredness (he used 'tiredness' and 'lack of motivation' synonymously) needed some attention. Michael had sought advice from several health professionals, yet he felt that he was largely unheard and unhelped. Tiredness and the consequent difficulties in propelling the body into the world interfered with participants' abilities to work and to engage in recreational activities.

Tiredness and sleepiness are well-known side effects of neuroleptic medication and were recognised as such by several of the study participants. Judith found that her medication interfered with her ability to stay awake during the day, while Roger found that the sleepiness caused by his medication interfered markedly with his everyday life. He told me that he had asked for a reduction in his medication because his blood felt 'like concrete flowing in my veins'.

It is relatively easy to understand and sympathise with expressions of limitations because of tiredness or sleepiness. These are bodily experiences that have been shared to some degree by people who have never had a schizophrenic illness. However, the intense fear engendered by another side effect of antipsychotic medication, acute dystonic reaction,[2] is known only to those who have experienced it. As Lucy relates:

> *One of the big things that happened at school was they hadn't started giving me side-effect medication, side-effect pills. And my eyes turned up. Oh my God, that's the most . . . I've had that happen to me so many times when they've stopped giving me them. It's scary. You cannot sleep. You cannot close your eyes because they just blink so much. Oh I hate it. I wouldn't wish that upon my worst enemy. Your eyes creep to the ceiling. Oh God. You just can't bring them down. And you can't go to the toilet because you're too scared that you're going to keep looking up.*

ACCEPTING THE NEED TO TAKE REGULAR MEDICATION

Given the unpleasant side effects that were experienced by most of the study participants, it might not have been surprising to have found that the participants were reluctant to take medication. In fact this was not the case. While some were a little dubious about their need to take medication on a long-term basis, the general feeling expressed by all the participants was that medication was a necessity.

Most participants reported having considered carefully the consequences of not continuing with medication and felt that, on balance, it was better to tolerate troubling side effects than to risk the extreme distress associated with an acute episode of illness. Medication was thus a form of insurance, a way to help themselves stay well. Some were frustrated by the need to continue to take medication which so affected their functioning on a daily basis.

Of all the participants, Chris was the one most severely affected by medication side effects, to the extent that he regularly contemplated suicide:

> *Well it's . . . it's because of the side effects of the medication. Like I might have told you before it lowers my libido and that's why I want to kill myself. Just takes all the fun out of life. The only thing that makes adult life worthwhile and I no longer function properly at that level.*

There was a general acceptance among the participants in the study that their illness was a continuing and long-term one and that while some symptoms persisted, medication would be effective in enabling a return to a 'normal' life. Indeed, Simon even felt that he had been able to begin a *new* life once he had begun neuroleptic medication:

> *I think the time since I was put on antipsychotic drugs was the beginning of a new life . . . that it was gradually going downhill over the years through my teenage years. And I think . . . that a lot of the processes of adolescence occurred to me after that. After my . . . after the age of 25.*

In accepting their need to continue to take medication people with schizophrenia are faced with having also to deal with its side effects. In addition, the need to take medication signals that they are in some way different; although they appear well and wish to move on with their lives, they need protection from the possibility of further acute illness. Taking regular medication becomes a part of their Being-in-the-world.

COMING FACE TO FACE WITH THE MIND–BODY QUESTION

One of the greatest impacts that the experience of schizophrenic illness has on those who suffer from it, is on the way in which they find themselves contemplating the connection of mind and body. The process by which the person with schizophrenia comes to doubt his or her experiences is illustrated by Liz's statement that she did not initially doubt her experience of hearing voices, and that for some time she did not know that other people did not hear voices. Having come to this realisation, however, Liz now understands that nothing will ever be quite the same again:

> *Because you challenge your whole . . . every idea you have you challenge, because you think it could be, well you don't . . . at the time you don't think that it could be . . . but, as you get more insight, you think that your ideas could be psychotic in some way or, you know, or that they could be not like what other people are thinking . . . And you tend to question yourself quite a lot.*
>
> (Even when you're well?)
>
> *Oh yeah. But it's sort of at a less acute stage so you've got more time to think about it anyway. You're not sort of panicking. Yeah.*

Several other participants in the study also reflected on the effect that medication had had in changing their thoughts. To discover that one's beliefs might be changed by medication was to be challenged in a most fundamental and disturbing way. If my thoughts are able to be altered through some chemical intervention, then the question follows, 'Who am I?' Three statements that illustrate the participants' concern with this existential question are given below. The extract from Chris comes after his reference to persistent thoughts of suicide. As he explained, even these thoughts, which are regular, persistent and feel as if they are part of him*self*, might be made to leave:

> *But maybe Dr Mitchell will be able to change me. Like he's changing my medication and he might be able to change the way I think because until I had the last talk I had with him I always thought it would be ideal for me to be in a hospital and not on drugs, even if everyone else was not on drugs and they were all running round screaming and things like that I'd rather be like that because I'd be on a high. And he almost convinced me, well he's trying to convince me that even if I was on a high it wouldn't be good. And he's got a lot of knowledge about that sort of thing so I don't know. I'm having to rethink that and if you can make me rethink that you can make me rethink anything.* (Chris)

> *No, well, Dr Phillips has the opinion that . . . ah . . . you don't think what you think. You say I want to think this and so on but you don't actually do that. It's all automatic. Chemical, electrical. Take a pill and you think differently. Well it actually happens.* (Jack)

> *Experiences like that [the effect of medication in altering thought] can undermine one's confidence at the most profound level, I think. That you have such a graphic demonstration that one's own mind is a mechanism. That beliefs, which should have the validity of beliefs are really . . . can be changed by taking medication. That is a very difficult, a very deep thing to come to terms with.* (Simon)

Two other aspects of the mind–body connection are hinted at in these extracts: the effect of medication in controlling mood, and the location of thoughts and emotions in the brain. Chris spoke of his wish to be taken off medication even if he were then in need of hospitalisation, because he would be 'on a high'. Although, on the whole, participants would rather take medication than suffer the effects of illness, there was sadness expressed by several participants in that they felt 'controlled' by their medication. Drugs had the effect, they said, of limiting their feelings. They no longer felt strong emotions, either of sadness or of joy, and they missed experiencing these feelings. Liz described her experience in a way which was typical of several of the participants:

> *It's very confining, like you can never be really happy or really sad, you're just sort of in the middle, well that's how I feel. Really controlled. But you know sometimes you just feel like being really happy, but you can't be.*

To be controlled by medication is to lose part of oneself. Not only is a person in this situation faced with the question 'Who am I?' if chemical substances can change thoughts and beliefs, but if medication dampens emotions, people feel as if they are unable to express all of themselves. Liz feels that she would like to be happy but cannot be. She is unable to experience all she knows she could. She is unable to live up to the possibilities she sees and cannot express herself fully as who she is. In spite of its multiple effects, each participant accepted the 'trade-off', as Liz called it, of having to take medication on a long-term basis. The Being-in-the-world of the participants is affected by the chemicals they take in order not to suffer the symptoms of acute illness; at the same time the need and agreement to take medication is part of their Being-in-the-world.

Given the awareness of the connection between mind and body, it is not surprising that all of the participants at some stage spoke of schizophrenia as a problem located in the physical brain. Most spoke of schizophrenia as a brain disease or a chemical imbalance. One participant spoke of having lost his mind and another of his brain 'snapping'. This explanation of schizophrenia as located in the brain fits the experience of the participants and is not necessarily related to what the participants have read or been told, although it is compatible with some current theories of the cause of schizophrenia. The participants actually *experienced* brain problems rather than having learned or theorised that this is the 'real' nature of their illness.

Towards the end of the interview series, each of the study participants was asked to sum up what it was like for them to live with schizophrenia. The intensity of the experience for each of them and the effect that this illness has had (and does have) on Being-in-the-world are demonstrated in the two extracts which follow. Lucy spoke mostly about the feelings she had had when she was acutely ill; Liz carries her description into the present. Each of these women had felt dead during some of their illness. To feel dead while still alive is no longer to be a person at all, to have no place in the world. To feel dead while still alive is to be temporarily suspended in a place of nothingness. The whole of their Being was felt to be obliterated at least for a time. In their descriptions, there is a parallel with Chris's statement, cited earlier in this chapter, that he was for a time, 'in a living hell'. These feelings, along with those explained in the previous section, of 'one's mind as a mechanism', are deeply disturbing.

Lucy described a self-portrait which she painted in hospital:

> *This is just before I got shock treatment. I did this one in hospital. That's me. That's how I looked, honestly. The head and the heart. I never cried, never ever cried once in hospital. I just had no tears. I just felt so dead. And after the voices went I felt even less.*

When I asked Liz to sum up how having schizophrenia had changed her life, she said:

> *Six months of immobilisation. Yeah, literally, a period of being a dead person, for me anyway of achieving . . . well, for me not achieving anything . . . but, but in that respect too, it's sort of a period of rest too, I don't know . . . It's just being totally incapacitated, you know, like sort of being off the face of the earth, out in the black hole of Calcutta, in [hospital] not achieving anything, losing contact with people and . . . with experiences that you probably wouldn't have been through. Although my doctor says that I've actually learned quite a lot, and it's helped me in a big way, being schizophrenic . . . because he sees me as quite immature and . . . with a lot of insecurities and things, and that actually the schizophrenia has given me, or has been a big help to that. So, not that he knew me before I was schizophrenic.*

To be totally incapacitated, immobilised, a dead person, is to be completely overwhelmed. What could be more overwhelming than a living death? Yet out of this experience involving the loss and regaining of self, came growth and change; it was literally, a life-changing experience.

Nick's answer to the question 'What is it like to live with schizophrenia?' encompasses his life as a whole and powerfully sums up just how isolating it can be to have had so many experiences that others cannot share:

> *Oh I'd say it's . . . I'd say it's pretty hard, eh, because . . . I don't know . . . not everybody's made perfect in this world, you know, and not everybody's the same, you know, and I'd say that, you know, I'd say it's pretty hard living with schizophrenia because you're afraid that, you know . . . other people might think that you're a bit loopy or something, you know, eh? And I'd say that . . . I don't know . . .*

> *I'd say it's best just to do things that you believe in you know, and um . . . and just ignore what other people say, you know, and just . . . if they try to give you a hard time or something like that, you know, I just say . . . it's best to live your own life and don't let other people judge you if it's right or wrong, you know, because it's what you want to do, you know, so . . . I'd say it's best just to do things for yourself, you know, and just carry on what you're doing . . . I don't know . . . something like that.*

This is the way Nick *is*. While he recognises he is not perfect he has no choice; he is in-the-world in this way. Being-in-the-world means Being-with-others, a situation Nick finds difficult at times because of the way others treat him, the way he feels about them, and the advice and judgements which may be given to or about him. In this difficult situation, Nick finds it best just to be himself, to do what he believes to be right.

CONCLUSION

The discussion in this chapter has focused on the way in which people who suffer from schizophrenia experience their own Being-in-the-world. To have a schizophrenic illness means to have lived through at least one period of acute illness, to have in some way come to terms with a diagnosis, and to take medication on a continuing basis. Although schizophrenia is commonly understood to be a mental illness, it affects those who suffer from it in every dimension of their lives. Bodily, mental and emotional effects of the illness, and its subsequent treatment, have a profound impact on the sufferer's sense of self. While each person with schizophrenia goes about his or her life as a citizen, worker, parent and so on, they must do so against a backdrop of specific difficulties.

People with schizophrenia find themselves thrown into the world in a particular way. Each 'exists as an entity which has to be as it is and can be' (Heidegger 1927/1962, p. 321). Coming to terms with the realisation that one is unwell and reconceptualising one's Being-in-the-world in this light means in-corporating—taking into one's self—an image of oneself as Being-in-the-world in a new way. The distressing experiences of acute illness are followed by a deep and disturbing realisation that nothing will ever be quite the same again. Sufferers have to cope not only with an altered sense of bodily dwelling in the world, but they also find themselves occupied with thoughts to an extent which interferes with everyday activities.

Usually, in order to function effectively in the world, they must accept and continue to take medication which itself has unpleasant and hindering effects on their Being.

In addition to this, people with schizophrenia are faced with questions about the nature of existence. For most of us these belong to the philosophical realm, but for people with schizophrenia these questions stem directly from their experiences. Such questions centre on the nature of the connection between mind and body, and on the meaning of life if thoughts and beliefs can be changed through taking medication. The nature of 'thrownness' for a person with schizophrenia is such that it calls into question what it means *to be*, what it is to live life as a person-in-the-world.

Being-in-the-world also has other dimensions. To be-in-the-world means to be-with-others. Others form a substantial part of the world into which we are thrown; we interact with others on a daily basis, but we are also part of a social and cultural ethos which has developed over time. Finding themselves in the world in the way outlined in this chapter, schizophrenia sufferers must engage in activities in which others are involved, and live in the world alongside others.

The participants in the study went about their lives with strength and courage. They managed themselves well in the face of ongoing illness through careful planning, pacing themselves and monitoring their thoughts and actions. Understanding and accepting the nature of their illness, and recognising that care is needed in managing their lives from here on have enabled most of the participants to integrate their past into their present. In doing so they are each able to recall their past, to recognise and come to terms with that experience and to let it go. They avoid dwelling on their illness or the past, yet continue with life in the light of the understanding they have from these experiences, which are part of who they are-in-the-world. It is not only the participants themselves who must let go; family and health professionals must learn to accept them as no longer unwell, and to let go of the 'patient' or 'sick' ways in which they were previously known.

Managing life with a chronic illness means that one must be able to recall what things were like, yet proceed onwards with life in spite of the pain and difficulties of the past. The profound experiences which comprised their illness, coupled with an often less than sympathetic social world, led each of the participants to take a clear stand on their own values and to rely on themselves. Knowing that they were in many ways removed from others by virtue of the experiences they had undergone, each has made choices that lead in the direction they themselves wish their lives to go. As researcher, my continuing impression of the study participants is of a group of strikingly different individuals, each with his or her own desires, wishes and ambitions. It is my belief that good nursing care for people with a schizophrenic illness rests fundamentally on our ability to recognise people's individual needs and work with them towards achieving their own goals, hopes and dreams.

NOTES

1. Chris has made an intentional pun here. The nurse's name in the book and film is Nurse Ratched.
2. An acute dystonic reaction is characterised by abnormal, sustained posturing movements of the neck, jaw and eyes. It often involves protrusion of the tongue, spasms of jaw muscles and oculogyric crisis.

REFERENCES

Aldiss, B.W. 1990 'Introduction: Kafka's sister' *My Madness: The Selected Writings of Anna Kavan* ed. B.W. Aldiss Pan Books, London, pp. vi–xiv

Bachrach, L.L. 1988 'Defining chronic mental illness: a concept paper' *Hospital and Community Psychiatry* vol. 39, no. 4, pp. 383–8

Barham, P. & Hayward, R. 1991 *From the Mental Patient to the Person* Routledge, London

Dostal, R.J. 1993 'Time and phenomenology in Husserl and Heidegger' *The Cambridge Companion to Heidegger* ed. C. Guignon Cambridge University Press, Cambridge, pp. 141–69

Godschalx, S.M. 1989 'Experiencing life with a psychiatric disability' *Chronic Mental Illness: Coping Strategies* ed. J.T. Maurin Slack, Thorofare, N.J., pp. 3–29

Hall, H. 1993 'Intentionality and world: division I of Being and Time' *The Cambridge Companion to Heidegger* ed. C.B. Guignon Cambridge University Press, Cambridge, pp. 122–40

Heidegger, M. 1927/1962 *Being and Time* (trans. J. Macquarrie & E. Robinson) Basil Blackwell, Oxford

Kleinman, A. 1988 *The Illness Narratives* Basic Books, New York

Leary, J., Johnstone, E.C. & Owens, D.G.C. 1991 'Social outcome' *British Journal of Psychiatry* vol. 159 (suppl. 13), pp. 13–20

Morse, J.M. & Johnson, J.L. 1991 'Toward a theory of illness: the illness constellation model' *The Illness Experience* eds J.M. Morse & J.L. Johnson Sage, Newbury Park, Ca., pp. 315–42

Packard, N.J., Haberman, M.R., Woods, N.F. & Yates, B.C. 1991 'Demands of illness among chronically ill women' *Western Journal of Nursing Research* vol. 13, no. 4, pp. 434–57

Sass, L.A. 1992 *Madness and Modernism: Insanity in the Light of Modern Art* Basic Books, New York

Schooler, N.R. 1994 'Negative symptoms in schizophrenia: assessment of the effect of risperidone' *The Journal of Clinical Psychiatry* vol. 55, no. 5 (suppl.), pp. 22–8

Stewart, D. & Mickunas, A. 1974 *Exploring Phenomenology* American Library Association, Chicago

Torrey, E.F. 1988 *Surviving Schizophrenia* Harper & Row, New York

Vellenga, B.A. & Christenson, J. 1994 'Persistent and severely mentally ill clients' perceptions of their mental illness' *Issues in Mental Health Nursing* vol. 15, pp. 359–71

Walton, J.A. 1995 *Schizophrenia: A Way of Being-in-the-World* unpublished PhD thesis, Massey University, Palmerston North, New Zealand

WHO Scientific Group on the Treatment of Psychiatric Disorders 1991 *Evaluation of Methods for Treatment of Mental Disorders* WHO Technical Report Series 812, WHO, Geneva

seven

On living with chronic pain

ANN O'LOUGHLIN

This chapter addresses the experience of chronic pain. The study on which it is based was unusual in that only one participant was involved. As the author demonstrates, the phenomenological case study involving only one participant is both feasible for the researcher and enlightening for the reader.

Data for the study were collected during a series of conversational dialogues. In order to protect the participant several details of her story have been disguised, and the name used is fictional. We ask that all readers appreciate that the most horrific details of the story have actually been watered down in our effort to safeguard Ana's anonymity. Nevertheless, we believe that the essence of Ana's story remains, and that the important lessons to be learned from it are still to be found in this chapter.

The study on which the chapter was based was conducted as part of a postgraduate Diploma in Social Science (Nursing).

ACROSS CULTURES AND across time pain is one of the most basic human experiences. The meaning of pain is embedded in the underlying beliefs of the culture in which it is situated. In contemporary Western society pain is commonly viewed in a dichotomised way, as either physical or mental. From this viewpoint physical pain is seen as accompanying a broken arm and mental pain a broken heart.

Pain is often further classified as either acute or chronic, and chronic pain as either malignant or non-malignant in origin. The focus of the present study is on chronic pain of non-malignant origin. Such pain often has no obvious physiological cause and no cure. Unlike acute pain which is short-lived and functional, chronic pain is unrelenting, persisting long after it can serve any useful function (Melzack & Wall 1988).

Chronic pain is acknowledged as one of the most pervasive and expensive healthcare problems today (Hitchcock et al. 1994). It all too often encompasses every aspect of a person's life 'with resultant moral, social and financial implications for society' (Carroll & Bowsher 1993, p. 51). In a comparative study across cultures Kodiath and Kodiath (1989, cited in Kodiath 1991) describe the loneliness, depression and hopelessness people felt as a result of chronic pain. Unlike acute pain—which subsides as healing takes place, is usually relieved by analgesic medication and has a predictable end—chronic pain is highly complex, occurs almost daily over many months and even years, and often does not respond to currently available methods of pain relief (McCaffery & Beebe 1989).

Healthcare professionals generally have inadequate knowledge of the complexities of the experience of chronic pain. Although clinical practice in this field is changing to some degree there is still evidence that chronic pain is not being managed as well as it could be. Many practitioners still manage chronic pain in a similar way to acute pain, with the primary treatment being pharmacological (Owens & Ehrenreich 1991). However, pharmacological management alone is seldom the total answer to the problem of chronic pain. As a result drug dosage is often raised progressively to the point at which significant side effects occur (NIH Consensus Development Conference 1987). This has the effect of leaving patients feeling frustrated and angry.

Considerable medical research has been done into the problem of chronic pain. Most of this research concentrates on individual factors in the sufferer and on changes in pain as a result of various combinations of interventions. As a nurse my interest in this study was to examine not pain itself, nor the ways in which pain may be controlled, but rather what it is like to experience chronic pain—what it is to be a person in pain. Gullickson (1993) conducted a Heideggerian hermeneutic analysis of the lived experience of persons with chronic illness; apart from this, at the time of my study, no similar investigation of lived experience of persons with chronic pain could be located. To understand human experience from the individual's perspective fits well conceptually with a nursing perspective, which aims to more fully grasp the patient's definition (perception) of an event or experience (Davis 1973).

My interest in the phenomenon of chronic pain arose initially from my father's experience of living with the chronic pain of osteoarthritis since young adulthood. It was reinforced during my nursing career, in particular as a student nurse and newly registered nurse, when I failed to find adequate solutions to the problems faced by patients experiencing chronic pain. Nursing interventions, both then and now, are generally limited by rigid adherence to options sanctioned by the medical model. These options (mostly pharmacological) frequently offer no more than limited relief to individuals in chronic pain.

The American nurse scholar Afaf Meleis has observed that 'the more ways in which we can analyze any phenomenon, the more potential there is for seeing different images and details that are not readily apparent when only viewed from one perspective' (1991, p. 249). Thus there is value in examining chronic pain from the person's perspective, a perspective not often considered.

The research approach for the present study was based largely on the writings of van Manen (1990), who combines the ideas of several phenomenological philosophers (including Heidegger, Husserl and Merleau-Ponty) to develop a hermeneutic phenomenological research approach. The approach is further influenced by the interpretation by Leonard (1994) of Heidegger's phenomenological view of person.

Phenomenological philosophy fits well with the one-participant approach used in this study. Davidson (1994), in referring to Husserl, believes that phenomenology has taught us that although each act of experiencing is unique to an individual, 'the meanings of this experience transcend both the subject and the intentional act' (1994, p. 210). Therefore when the past experiences of one person are grasped they may also relate to the 'lives of many others who have had similar experiences' (Davidson 1994, p. 211). By uncovering the essence of one woman's experience of living with chronic pain we can consider the insights gained in relation to the lives of others who are living with this problem.

THE STUDY PARTICIPANT

The participant in this study, Ana, is a middle-aged Caucasian woman who has lived with chronic pain since the age of three. Ana is married and has three adult children who live away from home. In recent years Ana has been diagnosed as having fibromyalgia.

Fibromyalgia can be described as a syndrome, the main feature being chronic painful muscles for which no definitive physiological changes can be detected (Schaefer 1995). Persons with fibromyalgia are affected to varying degrees. Symptoms include widespread, inexplicable pain; decreased pain threshold; fatigue; sleep disturbance; stiffness; psychological distress; and other symptoms such as headache, irritable bladder, irritable bowel and subjective swelling (Wolfe 1995). Ana has most of these symptoms.

The aetiology of fibromyalgia has not been established, and according to Wolfe the syndrome still needs to be defined clearly. Most discussions in medical literature focus to some extent on whether fibromyalgia is a psychological disorder, a physical disorder or a combination of both (e.g. Cohen et al. 1995; Russell 1995; Wolfe 1995).

DATA COLLECTION

Data were collected during three audiotaped dialogues and in informal discussions over coffee (as researcher I then documented impressions in a diary). The term 'dialogue' is used here rather than 'interview' as it better reflects my involvement as researcher in the research process and 'recognizes the shared experiences we have with other people as an important source of new knowledge' (Walters 1994, p. 140). This view is supported by other contemporary phenomenological researchers including van Manen (1990), although he uses the term 'conversational interview' rather than dialogue.

During my initial meeting with her, Ana informed me that she was about to undergo counselling for sexual abuse. We discussed the appropriateness of her participation in the study at this time and it was agreed that she would discuss this with her counsellor. After doing so Ana informed me that she still wished to take part in the study. Her ongoing participation was reviewed by both of us before each subsequent session.

Anonymity is an important ethical issue in a one-participant study as all the data in the final study report relate to the one person. Care has been taken not to include aspects of the participant's story which are most likely to identify her. At the time of the study many aspects of Ana's experiences that were included in the initial study report were known only to herself, her husband, her counsellor and myself. This increased the likelihood that anonymity would be maintained.

Given the time elapsed since the original study, and the possibility that some of this information might now be known more widely, the editors of this collection have also changed some details in a further attempt to maintain Ana's anonymity.

ANA'S STORY

Ana's story needs to begin at the beginning of her life because that is the beginning of her pain. To understand her pain you need to hear her story.

Ana explained this to me during our first dialogue together. As she began to tell me her story, she paused and asked, 'Is this what you want?' I replied: 'What I want is to hear about your experiences of living with chronic pain. Is that what you are telling me?' Ana wasted no time in reassuring me (she needed no reassurance herself) that indeed what she was relaying to me was her story of living with chronic pain. 'It is all part of it,' she said.

As Ana told me the story of her life, I was taken along on her journey and at the same time I experienced a journey of my own. At times her story connected with my story as a person, a woman, a mother, a nurse, and the daughter of a man who lives with chronic pain. At the same time her story was separate from mine in that her life experiences were different and unique. Listening to her I experienced a range of emotions, including sadness, anger and a growing sense of awe at Ana's courage and stoicism in the face of her traumatic life experiences. At times we laughed together as we shared stories of amusing life experiences.

Phenomenology is about uncovering essences and the following poem written by Ana captures the essence of her story and her need to relay it. Central to Ana's experience is the feeling that she has seldom been heard. The art of listening is integral to both phenomenological research and to nursing practice. Without listening there cannot be understanding and acceptance of the person as a situated being. In her poem, Ana voices her need to be listened to, heard and accepted for who she is. The last lines reflect her courage to carry on, which will also be demonstrated in the story that follows the poem.

Acceptance

Listen to me

Listen to me
From
morning to night

daylight to dusk
moans to groans
twists to turns
fears to tears
pain to prayers
chaos to crisis

give it a rest

change the software
Dear Lord

then a stranger I would be
that would not be me

I can still see the dewdrops
Praise God

I invite you, the reader, also to listen to Ana's story, below, so that you too might gain some insight from her experiences. Ana's experiences will be both similar to and different from the experiences of other sufferers of chronic pain. I hope that these similarities and differences will trigger insights for you as they have for me.

Ana's story is organised under themes which have been chosen as representing the essence of her experiences. The first theme 'My past life is my present pain' is significant in that it is the background essence of her story. The other themes identified include:

- being in a body of pain;
- living with fear, isolation and difference;
- being labelled and seeking validation;
- striving for control and surviving the pain; and
- uncovering patterns and learning to live.

My past life is my present pain

Ana begins her story at the age of three, describing the family with whom she lived as her mother, father and older sister. She identifies this time as the beginning of her experience of pain (and *sickness*), a time when she first experienced sexual and physical abuse by her father. Ana's mother was unaware of the abuse.

> *My mother was in the hospital and that was the first time I knew what sexual abuse was about . . . and I can't, I can't even begin to tell you what it was like because my father also tried to kill me at that time [her father pushed her violently into the sea in a fit of rage] and I suddenly felt that there was something very wrong with me, you know, and I couldn't get it together, and it was after that that I first*

knew what pain was about. I got sick, felt sick and I had pains in my legs and my stomach and I had high temperatures.

The pain and sickness continued through her childhood and resulted in interrupted patterns of schooling, a lack of friendships and severe isolation. At one stage Ana spent two years in bed and at other times she would attend school for two days in a week and then have six months off. Despite her poor attendance at school Ana strove to be the best at everything she did and was top of her class.

The family doctor used to visit on Saturdays, and at one stage Ana was admitted to hospital for tests, however no diagnosis was made of her condition. Neighbours visited and asked what was wrong but nobody seemed to know. Ana herself did not know what was wrong with her and found her illness difficult to understand.

The abuse of Ana by her father continued in her teenage years; at this time her parents were divorcing:

As a teenager . . . when my family was breaking up and my mum and dad divorced and . . . I had been abused then . . . and more importantly my dad tried to sell me [to one of his acquaintances] . . . and I have never forgotten that. But at that point in time was when I was becoming a teenager and that was robbed from me [normal teenage development].

Ana was pregnant at the age of fifteen, married and had two children by the age of eighteen. Married life was difficult for her. Ana's husband was an 'entrepreneur' and Ana worked all night in his factory, the children sleeping there while their parents worked. When Ana's eldest son was a toddler, two-thirds of his body was burnt in an accident. When he came home from hospital he would sleep only for twenty minutes at a time and this sleeping pattern lasted until he was three years old. Severe sleep deprivation and ongoing pain led to Ana becoming depressed:

My husband dragged me along to a psychiatrist because I was crying all the time. I was crying all the time [quietly]. And he said, 'But it's not normal to cry all the time.' And I looked at him and I thought 'no' . . . I was eighteen, unhappily married, two young children, one who had been severely burnt, worked all night in a factory, had no money, no electricity, migraine after migraine, severe sleep deprivation, was constantly drugged and doped and a few other minor matters, like my mother being seriously ill, and . . . it was not normal to cry in such circumstances [laughs].

Physical pain and sickness continued throughout Ana's adult life. She described leg pains, stomach pains and migraines, and although the pain (and her life) had its ups and downs the migraines in particular caused a lot of suffering. Her ability to cope with the pain was closely related to her life's circumstances at the time.

Ana's journey continued through two more marriages and several incidents of physical, sexual and emotional abuse. At times she suffered severe financial hardship as she balanced sole-parenting, employment and coping with the pain and the disability it caused.

Throughout her adult life Ana had several consultations with physicians for gynaecological problems, psychiatrists for depression, and a variety of other doctors to seek answers to her pain. She was prescribed a variety of drugs, developed addictions to many of them and subsequently went through withdrawal. Today she takes medications for hypertension but takes no medications for pain. While addicted to drugs she attempted suicide twice and on one occasion had shock treatment [electroconvulsive therapy] for depression.

In recent years Ana has been diagnosed with fibromyalgia, has attended a chronic pain management program with some benefits and is a member of a support group from which she gains much needed support. At the time of this study, Ana was living with her third husband, attending church regularly and having weekly counselling sessions for past sexual abuse.

Being in a body of pain

Intermingled with Ana's story of her life were clear descriptions of the pain that she felt in her body and how her body reacted to that pain. As can be seen from the following quote the body pain was closely related to, and indeed inseparable from, the emotional pain and other embodied reactions. Ana describes the pain she experienced during her childhood:

> *I remember the high temperatures, always being hot and then being very, very cold. And the thing I remember most of all, the pain in my stomach and my legs and always this clenching and trying to get away from it . . . you know . . . pain in my legs more than anything . . . pain in my legs, and . . . just the fact that whenever I tried to do anything . . . like if I tried to do anything I would always feel sick. No matter what I tried to do I would feel sick.*

Ana's pain was worse at night, and was closely related to a feeling of not being safe in bed:

God, I can remember the nights were horrific. I used to twist and turn and I still do that . . . this clenching and trying to get away.

This embodied response to the pain continues to this day and is not understood by Ana:

I don't know why I think it will help but it's a constant thing to relax my muscles at night because I fight them. I can control them in the daytime but at night my legs clench, my teeth clench, my hands . . .

Although the intensity of body pain varied according to what was happening in Ana's life at the time, she described her pain as always there. The degree of pain affected her level of functioning, and the level of functioning in turn affected how she coped with the pain. The inability of the body to function effectively was often more difficult than the actual pain. Ana expressed severe frustration at the limitations her body put on her life, frequently referring to her body as 'a pain in the neck'. Ana's frustration with her body is demonstrated in the following statement:

You feel this trap . . . you're trapped, you're trapped, you're trapped by your body. Your body is a pain in the neck and I feel as if I'm trying to get out of concrete . . . that I'd just like to break it open.

Ana has lived with pain for so long that she cannot imagine herself without the pain:

What would I do without the pain? You know you have to ask yourself that sometimes.

Ana does not mean that she does not want to be free of the pain but that the pain is such an integral part of her being that she has difficulty imagining herself without it.

Living with fear, isolation and difference

Ana experienced fear and isolation throughout her life. This fear and isolation was a significant part of her overall pain experience. During my first interview with Ana, when I needed reassurance that the focus of her discussion was indeed her experience of living with chronic pain, I asked her a specific question:

(Ana, how would you describe the pain at that stage?)

That I was aware of as a kid?

(Yes)

> *I didn't feel safe. That's the first thing. We had a house that had a verandah across the front of it and the room that I had was virtually just the width of a bed and a passage way. And they put a little partition and a curtain for a door which was virtually open to the outside. And of course with the fear that I had of my father and the guns and that I was never safe . . . So I had a feeling of not being safe in bed. And my bed should have been a haven from the world . . . if you can understand.*

Ana was brought up as a Catholic, and because she blamed herself for the abuse by her father she had a terrible fear that she 'wasn't going to go to heaven'. To cope with her fear she strove to be the best at everything she did. This trait, however, contributed to her isolation as it separated her even further from the other children, who named her 'Miss goody-goody'. Today Ana interprets her childhood striving for perfection as a reaction to fear:

> *It wasn't that I wanted necessarily to be the best. It was that I was too scared to do anything wrong . . . It was like fear . . . There was this little girl who was terrified. I had to do everything right.*

Being the 'only Catholic child in the street' contributed to Ana's isolation, as did the lack of contact with other children resulting from her erratic attendance at school:

> *You know I might only go to school two days a week. And that carried right through. I'd be there for a bit, then I'd have six months off and I always had this always being sick. And from having the leg pain, then I got the stomach pains, then I got the migraines. And that was sort of like from age five to thirteen . . . that was the pattern.*

The feeling of isolation remained with Ana throughout her adult life as she strove, often as a sole parent, to make a living, bring up her three children and cope with the pain and sickness. Friends (and husbands) came and went, and for a large part of her adult life she lived in a city where there were no relatives on whom she could call for support.

> *The memory I have of this was the total rejection . . . you know the feeling of how bad you are when you can't cope with life . . . and I don't know . . . just the memory that I have of it is just always being alone . . . and somebody going.*

Adding to her feeling of isolation and difference was the labelling she experienced by healthcare professionals and others.

Being labelled while seeking validation

Ana believed that explicit or implicit labels have been applied to her in relation to her health status since an early age. The underlying meaning implied in such labels had a significant effect on her perception of herself and on the way she believed she was perceived by others. The labels she believed most commonly applied to her were 'sick', 'chronic pain patient' and 'psychiatric' or 'ex-psychiatric patient'.

Ana recalled many incidents throughout her adult life that have contributed to this belief that she was labelled or stereotyped. She was first aware of being labelled at the age of eighteen, when she was diagnosed with depression. Although she believes now that her depression was related to her social situation as well as to her unrelenting pain, rather than to any underlying psychiatric illness, she was at that time referred to a psychiatrist for treatment:

> *At this time people were starting to say . . . and I was starting to get this lovely history of labels . . . labels . . . mental . . . nutcase.*

Many health professionals also implicitly labelled her. Ana believes that once these professionals knew her medical history, the overriding impression they had of her was as a chronic pain patient or as an ex-psychiatric patient, rather than having any impressions of her as a person. The assumption underlying these labels is that pain 'is in the head' and therefore not real, not valid or else the fault of the sufferer.

Implied labelling also affected the treatment she received for health-related problems not associated with her chronic pain condition. Ana gives an example:

> *If I went to the doctors with a broken ankle, they would give me valium. It doesn't matter what is wrong with you once you are labelled either with depression or chronic pain it will always affect the way doctors look at you.*

The interrelationship between the effects of labelling and Ana's failure to find healthcare professionals who would validate her as a person are highlighted in the following anecdote.

Ana recalled experiencing chest pain and difficulty breathing while driving home one day. The pain was unfamiliar and she began to wonder whether it was related to her heart, so she reluctantly drove herself to the Accident and Emergency Department of a large hospital. When she told the receptionist she had chest pain the response was immediate. All the usual procedures for checking out chest pain were commenced. However this came to a rapid halt when her file arrived:

My file had finally been collected. And what do I hear? A couple of nurses saying to the sister in charge, 'Have you seen her file?' The next minute I get the sister coming in: 'You can't take up this bed all day.' Virtually 'on your trolley' . . . Now I don't know if anybody knows what that feels like but it feels like shit.

To Ana, validation means having health professionals who listen, reassure, and 'make sure there is nothing new'. She is aware that there is usually nothing anyone can do for her pain but:

I get to the stage where my commonsense tells me I must just go [and get the symptoms checked out] . . . I'm not asking for drugs. And nobody says to me great, you're coping. You know, 'You're coping.' Nobody ever says that to you—that you are doing OK. You know, I feel I have to check some things out . . . and it's a pain.

Today Ana reluctantly attends a family doctor for management of hypertension, and avoids any discussion of her pain unless she is specifically asked how she is doing. To explain this attitude, Ana gave an example of a recent visit to her GP. As she was about to leave the GP's office, the doctor asked her how she was doing. Ana gave her 'a quick summary of what's been going on in my life'. Following this summary:

Jan [the doctor] said to me 'you know everyone over 40 has aches and pains', and she said 'you can't let it get you down'. And I thought 'I don't believe this' [angrily]. It shook me . . . I felt as if I was being treated like a child and I felt ghastly about it. I was speechless . . . and it didn't really do anything. It didn't support me, it didn't really help me as her patient, and it didn't really achieve anything. All it did was to dismiss it and it certainly didn't acknowledge that she believed or knew what the chronic pain condition was about.

The support and validation that Ana seeks is coupled with an understanding of the difficulties faced by her family:

When you're always in pain, you're a pain to every other bloody person around you . . . My husband often tells me that when you've got chronic pain, you are a chronic pain. He's not trying to be nasty. It's just that that's what it's like to live with someone who has pain all the time.

Striving for control and surviving the pain

For Ana striving for control has meant attempting to live a normal life while coping with pain. 'Balancing' and 'juggling' were terms she frequently used to describe how pain, life activities and stresses had to be dealt with simultaneously. I originally suggested to Ana a theme of coping with pain, but Ana emphasised that for most of her life she survived rather than coped. It is only in more recent years that she has managed to begin to 'tip the scales' more in the direction of living or coping.

From childhood on, Ana's poor health and the stressful circumstances in her life significantly affected her ability to cope:

> *I couldn't cope with school and a lot of what I did and what happened was literally because I couldn't deal with having to actually physically cope with my health and with the circumstances in my life, and go to school.*

Surviving the pain for Ana involves accommodating everyday activities as much as possible and gaining sufficient rest so that the pain is kept within tolerable limits. To Ana juggling and balancing means the difference between her controlling her life and the pain controlling her:

> *That [balancing life activities to accommodate the pain] took quite a lot of years . . . to accept that, for me, I couldn't live life in the fast lane . . . and at that time I was still trying to earn an income and that didn't work for me because I was always sick or I had too much pain and things would happen. And there were too many things going on in my life. And trying to look after kids and trying to have a social life. And it wasn't really until I accepted that I couldn't do that, that I was able to get the migraines down to some normality.*

Life however is often unpredictable, and Ana frequently experiences situations that result in extra stress and physical activity and that tip the balance too far. This results in increased pain and depression and affects her ability to cope. For Ana the effect of the pain on her life is more difficult to accept than the sensation of pain itself:

> *I want to be able to control and change my life and do what I want to do every day . . . like if I decide to wake up in the morning and go for a picnic or to the pictures tonight or go out to dinner . . . I can't do it. I can't do those things . . . Well I can do them but I might be in bed for weeks afterwards . . . and there's a frustration that builds*

up inside you because I feel that I'm controlled all the time . . . and that will make me do things that I know I'm going to pay for . . . you know . . . what's going to control you? The pain? Or you? . . . but if you just ignore it you're in trouble.

Ana believes that her life has been a matter of coping and surviving, 'living from minute to minute', and 'shutting out a lot of things that are happening'. She lives with the loss of what could have been possible had she had a 'normal', functioning body. She describes the pain as always being present and has to adjust her activities around her level of functioning and the pain in her body. Clearly there are times when the pain is worse than others:

There is always with pain you have your ups and downs . . . and you wax and wane . . . and depending on what's happening in my life at that time there have been times in my life when it's not been so bad.

Striving for control means that Ana has developed some techniques to assist her to control her pain without medication. Ana stopped taking medication for pain several years ago when she realised that she was taking more and more and not gaining relief. She described herself as having been addicted to many medications and found the side effects worse that the pain itself. Today she uses relaxation and visualisation techniques as aids to controlling pain:

With relaxation and visualisation I always have this other place. In this other place there is a waterfall and a beach and I can float above myself, look down on myself, and separate myself from the pain.

Ana's spiritual beliefs are also a source of strength to her. Although she stopped going to church during her teenage years 'because my parents were divorced'[1] she still believes in God. Ana described one significant spiritual experience she had during a particularly low time in her life:

I don't view this as some great evangelical experience but there certainly was an experience . . . and it started at this point because I was so cold. One of the things I have always had are these extremes of temperatures, which started way back when I was in bed for those years. And a lot of that cold experience and hot experience is like when I've been drowned [a reference to the attempted drowning in childhood]. And all of a sudden it was sort of like coming into light and the memory I have is of being in the dark and then coming into light . . . and then finally becoming warm. And it was at that instant that I knew I wasn't alone. I don't pretend to say I suddenly believed in God or anything

> *else but what I think happened to me then was that I was suddenly aware of my own spirituality to the extent that I had some resource I could draw on.*

Uncovering patterns and learning to live

Ana has been seeking understanding of and answers to her pain throughout most of her life. She found it difficult not knowing what was wrong and believed that she was to blame for the abuse by her father. She did not relate her sickness to the abuse. The possibility of these links was suggested to Ana recently and this knowledge has led her on a new journey.

Ana was taken down several 'treatment pathways' as an adult. They resulted in a range of outcomes from minimal relief to iatrogenic problems. As she has progressed through her life she has developed an embodied understanding of herself and her health problems which often conflicts with the interpretation and subsequent management that healthcare professionals instigate. Ana actively seeks any new information about her condition and is always interested in the latest medical research:

> *I accept that genetically . . . I accept quite categorically that genetically the temperament that you are can be a factor in having pain and the way you react to it . . . but that's just the beginning . . . it's only the beginning.*

Several months before I met Ana she had become aware of the possible links between sexual abuse and chronic pain syndrome. Although there was initial fear and anxiety about having to go down another pathway and uncover another painful aspect of life she bravely sought counselling. Ana more recently told me that the process of telling her story for this study was one of the major turning points in her healing process. It enabled her to begin uncovering the patterns that she now identifies as being significant in contributing to her gradually improving health status. This is how she describes the beginning of this journey:

> *The biggest thing to me at the moment is: I am middle-aged and I feel that I'm starting to have to learn to live. You know I have lived so long with the thought that I should be dead and it's such a new concept to me that I actually don't know how to live, even though I've lived all this time and done all these things. And I feel quite strange about that . . . you know . . . Because my life has been a matter of coping and surviving I don't know how to change gear to suddenly do the*

things I want to do because I really haven't known myself. I've only known the pain and the effort.

Part of Ana's learning to live involves her maintaining control of her life and her activities. Recently she became aware of the controls that others have placed on her throughout her life. She has felt controlled by her father, past husbands, doctors and many other people who surreptitiously placed demands on her. Ana has developed a level of assertiveness which means that she refuses many requests and, although she realises that she may offend many people in doing this, she also recognises that by monitoring her activities she can better control her pain (and her life).

PHENOMENOLOGICAL LIFEWORLD CONCEPTS AND THEIR MEANING FOR NURSING

The previous section has been presented in a way that will enable the reader to see the narrative nature of Ana's experience of living with chronic pain as well as the essential elements of her story as I have interpreted them. Clearly the themes as presented overlap and interrelate with each other. As can be seen from Ana's story, living with chronic pain is difficult, as is living with someone with chronic pain. Ana's world from an early age has had a significant impact on her way of being and the range of options that have been available to her. In turn Ana's way of being has had an effect on her world and the world of others around her.

In the following section I shall discuss Ana's story and argue that her way of Being-in-the-world was profoundly influenced by society's (including most healthcare professionals') dualistic notions of her as a person. Although this hegemonic view of a person is not changed easily, healthcare professionals and nurses in particular are challenged to view people using a more integrated mind–body approach. Phenomenological research and approaches to nursing care are seen as promoting different, more appropriate nurse–client relationships. This philosophical shift is particularly relevant in the approach to persons living with chronic pain or illness.

The French philosopher Descartes is commonly seen as being responsible for our current dualistic ideas about mind and body. For example, in Zohar (1990, p. 92) he is cited as saying:

> I rightly conclude that my essence consists in this alone, that I am a thinking thing . . . And although perhaps . . . I have a body with which I am closely conjoined, I have, on the one hand, a clear and distinct

> idea of myself as a thinking, non-extended thing, and on the other hand, a distinct idea of my body as an extended, non-thinking thing; it is therefore certain that I am truly distinct from my body, and can exist without it.

Although many people today would challenge Descartes' extreme view of mind–body separateness, this view still pervades our beliefs of what it means to be a person. Cassell (1982, cited in Benner & Wrubel 1989, p. 22) describes the effect such dichotomising has in relation to medicine's focus on problems of the body:

> If the mind–body dichotomy results in assigning the body to medicine, and the person is not in that category, then the only remaining place for the person is in the category of the mind. Where the mind is problematic (not identifiable in objective terms), its reality diminishes for science, and so too, does that of the person. Therefore, so long as the mind–body dichotomy is accepted, suffering is either subjective and not truly 'real'—not within medicine's domain—or identified exclusively with bodily pain. Not only is such an identification misleading and distorting, for it depersonalizes the sick patient, but is itself a source of suffering.

Chronic pain and chronic illness often become problematised under dualistic notions of person. These health problems do not fit comfortably into either the mind or the body domains. Rather, they tend to straddle these two categories: chronic pain/illness often is without any notable physiological cause and, at the same time, without sufficient evidence to put it clearly in the realm of the psychological. During Ana's childhood, physiological answers to the causes of her 'illness' were sought, however there appeared to be no recognition of, or attempt to uncover, any social, psychological or emotional factors. Cassell (1982) makes the point that the body is relegated to medicine; conversely it could be argued that if medical practitioners are consulted then 'bodily' answers to the problem will be sought. Many medical practitioners were consulted by Ana or her family throughout her life but it was not until recent years that links were made between her 'illness' and the abuse she experienced as a child.

From time to time throughout her adult life Ana's 'problem' was recategorised as a problem of the mind (still without any obvious links being made to her childhood abuse) and, as a consequence, Ana received treatment from psychiatrists including electroconvulsive therapy (ECT) and antidepressants. At the same time she and the medical doctors she consulted continued the search for physiological answers to her pain—it is clearly less problematic in our society if one's health problem is defined as having a physical rather than a psychological origin. It wasn't until Ana was well into mid-life and attended a chronic pain clinic that her pain problem was approached from a more integrated mind–body perspective, and she was helped to better understand the connection of mind and body in her particular situation.

Illnesses that lean towards the mind end of the spectrum (as some would suggest fibromyalgia does) and the people who suffer them are seen to be 'not truly real'. Ana had overwhelming impressions of being stereotyped negatively throughout most of her life with the result that she felt non-validated as a person. This stereotyping stemmed from her psychiatric history and from the implicit beliefs of some healthcare professionals that chronic pain originates from the mind and is therefore illegitimate. Clearly mind and body dichotomising by healthcare professionals created problems for Ana.

When healthcare professionals see their patients in such a divided way the patients are in a 'no-man's land', searching for a legitimate cause for their problems while battling the negative connotations of their psychiatric labels. This is how Ana perceives the problem:

> *If they [doctors] can't drug it out or cut it out, they literally don't know what to do. And that leaves you feeling as though you are just one big headache and a problem to everybody. And you get to the stage that you don't want to go to the doctor . . . I don't go to the doctor for years on end because of it.*

My analysis of the mind–body problem has focused here on medical literature because the healthcare professionals consulted by Ana were almost exclusively medical practitioners. Also most information on the subject of fibromyalgia is in the medical literature and nursing has its roots in medical science. Perhaps it is worthwhile reflecting here on the absence of reference to nurses in Ana's story. This is particularly significant in light of nursing's claim to 'holism' and the management strategies that people with chronic pain find useful. For Ana 'being listened to' was important, as was the education she received in relation to the development of skills such as pacing (balancing rest and activity), visualisation, biofeedback and relaxation techniques. These are all clearly education and pain management strategies that could be perceived as fitting a nursing approach, yet nurses were significant only in their absence from Ana's life.

Phenomenology, which challenges the Cartesian notion of mind–body separateness, puts forward the view that we are embodied rather than being minds that possess a body. According to Merleau-Ponty (cited in Moss 1978), one's body image is not pure knowledge based on reflection about the body. He believes that prior to reflection about the body, the individual forms a taken-for-granted familiarity with the body through everyday experiences: 'My body-image is built up around the immediate, pre-reflective familiarity with my own body, and with the network of actions possible for my body' (Merleau-Ponty, cited in Moss 1978, p. 77). This 'pre-reflective familiarity' is referred to by Benner and Wrubel (1989) as embodied intelligence. Because bodily functioning is mostly non-cognitive and 'automatic' it generally only comes to a person's awareness when something is wrong; that is, when everyday smooth functioning breaks down. According to Benner and Wrubel (1989), the loss of the habitual, skilled body makes the body feel foreign and objective, like a thing.

Aspects of Ana's story clearly indicate that she experienced loss of or disruptions to the habitual, skilled, functioning body as described above. Pain significantly affects smooth taken-for-granted functioning of the body as it causes movement to be noticed and modified to accommodate the pain. Unlike acute pain, which can usually be alleviated with analgesics, the nature of chronic pain is such that it is not easily relieved. Smooth everyday functioning is affected in an ongoing manner, forcing the person to find ways to adapt to the pain and incorporate it into their lifestyle. This is a significant challenge for all concerned—in particular the person with pain, but also family and healthcare professionals—and ought to be the focus of nursing practice. Nurses need to assist clients with chronic pain to regain a sense of control in their lives, rather than a sense of being controlled by the pain.

It is also essential that nurses (and other healthcare professionals) recognise the expertise of the person with the illness and the pain. These people live with pain from day to day and develop insights into their own body functioning, enabling them to make decisions based on their experience. Ana often receives negative messages from healthcare professionals when she wants to know more about drugs being prescribed or when she refuses them because of the negative side effects she has experienced in the past. Clearly her knowledge of her own body and how it reacts should be respected and taken into account when decisions about treatments are being made.

Ana's experiences of abuse as a child resulted in embodied responses. She recalled bodily reactions such as 'clenching', 'trying to get away', 'twisting and turning', and 'being able to control her muscles in the daytime but not at night'. Ana's responses can be seen as a reaction to her social and historical world, and as adaptive; the body recognises impending threats and danger before the nature of the danger is clear. However this adaptive capacity can also exert a toll. In Ana's case it is possible that her ongoing embodied anticipatory reactions to abuse have become maladaptive and are related to the chronic pain that she experiences today.

Ana's experience of living with pain in the present is very much related to her history. To know Ana in the present is to know her in the past. It is essential that we 'see' our clients in relation to their past lives. Otherwise we do not understand the possibilities available to them now or in the future. This is not a fatalistic attitude, rather it enables us to assist our clients with a degree of insight. Listening to Ana's story has given me a significant understanding of her present way of Being-in-the-world which I would not otherwise have had. In particular it has shown me the resilience and strength of character of a woman who has been subjected to significant stress and trauma throughout her life.

Ana's reflections on her past have enabled her to reinterpret aspects of her past in light of her current knowledge. Possible links between the abuse she was subjected to as a child and her present and past pain are currently being explored. Margaret Newman (1986), in her book *Health as Expanding Consciousness*, suggests that assisting clients to uncover significant patterns in their lives should be integral to nursing practice. She believes that pattern recognition provides insights which have the potential to influence health in a positive way. The dialogical approach used in my study contributed to Ana's pattern recognition at the same time as it enabled me to understand her in the present in relation to her past. Ana herself expressed great benefits from the approach. It is my belief, supported by Koch (1997), that the potential therapeutic effects of storytelling as a research approach have not yet been explored adequately.

Phenomenology allows us to view our world through 'different coloured glasses' and to see different possibilities. It supports an emphasis on the human response to health and illness in that it refocuses our attention on the concerns of the client. It does not ask that other perspectives be ignored but that they be perceived for what they are—a perspective only. Seeing a person through 'phenomenological glasses' is appropriate for nursing practice as it sets up possibilities for more humanistic interactions between nurses and clients. Such interactions are seen here as empowering for both clients and nurses and have the potential to positively influence the health of the client.

NOTE

1. The implication here is that because divorce is not sanctioned by the Roman Catholic church Ana would be ostracised.

REFERENCES

Benner, P. & Wrubel, J. 1989 *The Primacy of Caring: Stress and Coping in Health and Illness* Addison-Wesley, Ca.

Carroll, D. & Bowsher, D. 1993 *Pain: Management and Nursing Care* Butterworth-Heinemann, Oxford

Cohen, M., Sheether-Reid, R., Arroyo, J. & Champion, G. 1995 'Evidence for abnormal nociception in fibromyalgia and repetitive strain injury' *Journal of Musculoskeletal Pain* vol. 3, no. 2, pp. 49–57

Davidson, L. 1994 'Story telling and schizophrenia: using narrative structure in phenomenological research' *Humanistic Psychologist* vol. 21, no. 2, pp. 200–20

Davis, A. 1973 'The phenomenological approach in nursing research' *Doctoral Preparation for Nurses with Emphasis on the Psychiatric Field* ed. E. Garrison, University of California, San Francisco

Gullickson, C. 1993 'My death nearing its future: hermeneutical analysis of the lived experience of persons with chronic illness' *Journal of Advanced Nursing* vol. 18, pp. 1386–92

Hitchcock, L., Ferrell, B. & McCaffery, M. 1994 'The experience of chronic nonmalignant pain' *Journal of Pain and Symptom Management* vol. 9, no. 5, pp. 312–18

Koch, T. 1997 'Story telling: is it really research?' Inaugural Address, Flinders University, Adelaide

Kodiath, M. 1991 'Foreword' *Holistic Nurse Practitioner* vol. 6, no. 1, pp. 1–8

Leonard, V. 1994 'A Heideggarian phenomenological perspective on the concept of a person' *Interpretive Phenomenology: Embodiment, Caring and Ethics in Health and Illness* ed. P. Benner Sage, Thousand Oaks, Ca.

McCaffery, M. & Beebe, A. 1989 *Pain: Clinical Manual for Nursing Practice* Mosby, St Louis

Meleis, A. 1991 *Theoretical Nursing: Development & Progress* 2nd edn Lippincott, Philadelphia, Pa.

Melzack, R. & Wall, P. 1988 *The Challenge of Pain* rev. edn Penguin, London

Moss, D. 1978 'Brain, body, and world: perspectives on body-image' *Existential-Phenomenological Alternatives for Psychology* eds R. Valle & M. King Oxford University Press, New York

Newman, M. 1986 *Health as Expanding Consciousness* Mosby, St Louis

NIH Consensus Development Conference 1987 'The integrated approach to the management of pain' *Journal of Pain and Symptom Management* vol. 2, no. 1, pp. 35–41

Owens, K. & Ehrenreich, D. 1991 'Literature review of nonpharmacologic methods for the treatment of chronic pain' *Holistic Nurse Practitioner* vol. 6, no. 1, pp. 24–31

Russell, A. 1995 'Fibromyalgia: a historical perspective' *Journal of Musculoskeletal Pain* vol. 3, no. 2, pp. 59–65

Schaefer, K. 1995 'Struggling to maintain balance: a study of women living with fibromyalgia' *Journal of Advanced Nursing* vol. 21, pp. 95–102

van Manen, M. 1990 *Researching Lived Experience: Human Science for an Action Sensitive Pedagogy* Althouse Press, Ontario

Walters, A.J. 1994 'Phenomenology as a way of understanding in nursing' *Contemporary Nurse* vol. 3, no. 3, pp. 134–41

Wolfe, F. 1995 'The future of fibromyalgia: some critical issues' *Journal of Musculoskeletal Pain* vol. 3, no. 2, pp. 3–15

Zohar, D. 1990 *The Quantum Self: Human Nature and Consciousness Defined by the New Physics* Quill William Morrow, New York

eight

On inflicting and relieving pain

IRENA MADJAR

This chapter is based on a phenomenological study undertaken as part of a PhD in Nursing at Massey University in New Zealand. The aim of the original research was to describe the phenomenon of clinically inflicted pain—pain that is created in the process of nursing interventions. Such pain differs from pathological pain of disease or trauma since it has an external referent. It thus involves at least two persons: the one whose actions generate the pain, and the patient who must endure it. As described elsewhere (Madjar 1991; 1998) the study involved fourteen patients who had experienced burn injuries and who underwent dressing changes and other procedures in a burn care unit, or who were diagnosed with cancer and received intravenous chemotherapy in an oncology clinic. The study also included twenty nurses who provided direct care to these patients. In this chapter the focus is on one aspect of the original study—the discussion of how nurses working in a burn care unit experienced the challenge of inflicting and relieving pain in the course of their everyday work. This chapter is dedicated to the twenty nurses who allowed a researcher's gaze to be cast over their work and who teach us all that even among the pain there are possibilities for understanding, care and therapeutic partnership.

IN HIS CHAPTER earlier in this book, Max van Manen writes about the complementary natures of the gnostic act and the pathic hand, as well as the ambiguity between the pathic and gnostic touch employed in nursing practice. Nowhere is the tension between the two forms of touch more evident than in nursing acts that, regardless of the intent, involve the infliction of pain. Even conceptually it is not easy to distinguish between the 'gnostic' and the 'pathic', the technical and the empathetic, the 'instrumental' and the 'therapeutic' (Gadow 1984). In actual practice the similarities and the distinctions are not so much thought of as lived—sometimes with considerable difficulty for both those who inflict pain and those who must endure it.

Pain infliction is an inevitable part of the ordinary, everyday work of nurses in many clinical settings. Yet most are ill-prepared for this aspect of their work. In particular, as research by Fagerhaugh and Strauss (1977) has shown, the work of nurses in burn care units captures best the elemental nature of the nurse–patient encounter during which pain is inflicted and endured.

Patients who have suffered burns must undergo frequent, often daily, changes of dressings, cleaning of wounds and debridement—the cutting away and removal of dead and damaged tissue from the edges of the wound. Such dressing changes usually involve saline baths or showers to soak away soiled dressings and wound exudate, careful cleaning and drying of wounds, topical application of ointments and other medicaments, and re-dressing and rebandaging of the affected parts of the body. When burn injuries are extensive, such procedures can take one, two, or more hours. While the intent is to minimise risks of infection and scarring, and to aid healing, the process is often extremely painful for the patient and stressful for the nurse. Unlike the pain of disease which arises out of pathological processes within the body, this pain comes into being in the tactile encounter between the nurse and the patient. Despite the physical closeness during which this pain is generated, patients and nurses inhabit different lifeworlds and so apprehend inflicted pain from very different perspectives—it is the inherent uniqueness of human experience that makes it difficult for patients and nurses to share the experience in which they are so intimately involved. As so poignantly captured in the deceptively simple words of Elaine Scarry (1985, p. 13): 'To have pain is to have *certainty*, to hear about pain is to have *doubt*.'

The essential nature of the phenomenon of clinically inflicted pain has been described elsewhere (Madjar 1991; 1997; 1998)—the embodied certainty of the painfulness, its wounding nature, the handing over of one's body to others to wound and to hurt, and the need to restrain the body and the voice. Here the focus is on the experience of nurses and their perceptions of the tactile encounter which makes pathic presence possible. The focus is also on the doubt that separates nurses and patients and allows nurses to construct their patients' experiences in a different light from their own.

NURSES' EXPERIENCE OF PAIN INFLICTION

Since it is not their bodies which are handed over, wounded, hurt or restrained, nurses cannot physically experience the pain they are inflicting nor its impact on the embodied self of the patient. Indeed, it is *because* they do not feel the pain which the patient feels that nurses are able to perform procedures which patients experience as painful, and can be attracted to work in settings where pain infliction is a common part of their work. Yet, patients' experiences of pain are not totally private nor inaccessible, and so infliction of pain becomes a source of stress to nurses. If they were unaware of patients' suffering, then they would not feel a need to shield themselves from it. It is because they *do* sense something of patients' pain that nurses experience dis-ease and dis-comfort in performing procedures which, while clinically justified, are inherently painful. The instrumental aspect of the work of nurses can be satisfying personally and professionally, while at the same time giving rise to stress and concern.

It is significant that even though the study on which this chapter is based dealt only with adults, all the nurses interviewed brought up the subject of children and the stress of having to work with them. Nurses' perceptions of children as unable to appreciate the good intentions of staff, or to control their fears and emotional expressions were relevant for two reasons. First, adult patients were contrasted with children and the point made that, because they were not children, adults could be expected to respond to reasoning, information and verbal reassurance. Thus adult patients were expected to show composure, self-control and, above all, cooperation, irrespective of how painful the procedure or how much or how little pain relief had been provided. Second, the small number of adult patients who failed to live up to such expectations were considered to be immature in some way and, like children, beyond help by reasoning or by other rational means.

Overall, the nurses interviewed disliked inflicting pain and hurting patients in the process of treatment. Some speculated as to why a way had not been found to treat burn trauma without causing further pain and distress. However, pain control approaches—such as general anaesthesia, inhalation analgesia, patient-controlled analgesia and even continuous intravenous infusion of morphine or other opioids—were usually dismissed as impractical or involving too much risk for the patient. The nurses therefore considered that inflicting some pain was an inevitable part of their work, something new nurses had to accept and learn to do without being overwhelmed by patients' responses. Kate, a nurse with only five months' experience in the burn care unit described her feelings about performing procedures that are painful for the patient, and then contrasted her responses with how she sees more experienced nurses approaching their work:

> *I find that even after being here five months I tend to rationalise a lot of things, like the pain. I particularly found that the really hard thing to cope with when I first came here was the pain the patients were experiencing. And I used to think, 'Why can't I do something to stop this pain, why can't I give them an injection?' . . . It was really hard to get into thinking, 'This person is in pain, okay, fine. He'll be uncomfortable for the next twenty minutes while I do the dressing, but then he'll be all right.' . . . I don't like to cope with that myself, that I am inflicting pain so to speak, but I prepare myself by thinking, 'I'll get in there, I'll do it,' and in some cases detach yourself from the person for a time, while it hurts.*
>
> (How do you manage to do that? How do you achieve that detachment?)
>
> *I have to make a conscious effort to stop myself thinking, 'Oh look, you are hurting so and so.' I spend most of my time saying, 'I am really sorry. I don't mean to hurt you.' And I mean it. I am very sincere about it, but sometimes I have to think, 'Okay, this person is in pain, but I have to go ahead and do it.' . . . I just have to make a conscious decision to think, 'Get on with it!'*
>
> *The nurses who have been here [longer] are not hard, but their approach is different to mine. I've heard patients say, 'Nurse so and so, she's really rough.' It's not that they are rough, it's just that they can cope with the pain that the patient is undergoing at the time and just go ahead and do it, and not blink an eyelid, whereas I go in there and think, 'Oh no, they are in pain. I'll take my time,' and supposedly be more gentle . . . I can be more gentle and not get rid of all the air pockets [under a new graft] whereas they could be so called 'rough', get in there, clean it out, and be doing a thorough job, a better job than me . . . I sometimes feel very inadequate.*

This extract encapsulates several key issues that exemplify nursing practice and attitudes to the care of patients with burns: learning to accept the inevitability of pain rather than questioning its necessity in specific situations; learning to see pain as temporary and therefore of less consequence; learning to rationalise pain and teach oneself not to pay attention to it; learning to think that nurses are coping with patients' pain when they are able to ignore signs of pain and distress; learning that technical performance counts more than the amount of pain inflicted or avoided. All of these factors help to describe nurses' experience of being the ones who inflict pain and go on inflicting it. The interview extract also captures something of the ethos of the burn care unit in which this study was undertaken—the expectation that patients will endure their pain and be cooperative, and that nurses will ensure that regardless of how much pain their actions may cause, technical procedures will be done, and will be done thoroughly.

NURSES' PERCEPTIONS OF INFLICTED PAIN

If there is a paradox in what the burn care unit nurses considered to be the source of both stress and satisfaction in their work, there is also a paradox in how they perceived the pain generated through their work. Despite the visibility of patients' wounds and the directness of nurses' physical actions when providing wound care, many instances of patients' pain were not recognised, named or acknowledged as pain. Pain could be qualified, defined, explained or denied in such a way that it often became invisible and not real. Yet, overall, inflicted pain was difficult to ignore and it was perceived and presented to patients as largely inevitable and thus inescapably real, as well as non-harmful and even, by some nurses, as beneficial. These perceptions in turn resulted in the denial of pain in some instances and, in others, its interpretation as inevitable but of no great concern.

Visible and invisible pain

By definition all pain is invisible; it is a private experience which the person not in pain cannot know directly. Yet, relief of pain and suffering depends on this private experience being shared to the extent that a person's pain becomes another's concern, and thus acquires visibility and a social dimension. For pain to be made visible, it needs to be given voice, not only by the person in pain but also by those with the power to relieve it. Thus, making pain visible is a joint project which requires that the patient's body and voice are believed, rather than doubted or by-passed (Scarry 1985). In clinical practice, however, there are many ways of keeping pain private and invisible, thus denying or casting doubt on its facticity.

One way for nurses to recognise the reality of pain and make it visible is to anticipate it and prepare the patient adequately for it. In the burn care unit this happened when nurses acknowledged that certain circumstances would result in pain and acted accordingly. For example, pain was likely to be anticipated in relation to the first saline bath, debridement, the first change of dressings after skin grafting, or the premature removal of donor site dressings. In such situations, nurses were more likely to recognise the potential for pain, to provide some pain-relieving medication beforehand and to acknowledge patients' pain openly, sometimes apologising for actions that might have contributed to a patient's pain. The following extract from Tania's interview shows the reasoning and anticipation used with a particular patient:

> *I decided to give him intravenous morphine for his dressing to his hand because it is his first dressing. Because, based on past experiences, first dressings can be very painful, and intravenous morphine works much, much better than IM [intramuscular] morphine, much faster, and it just seems to control the pain so much better . . . Where you've had the skin laid it isn't going to be that painful. It's where there is no skin and you clean it and try to get off any debris, that is going to hurt. I think the object of a dressing is to get it done as swiftly and as efficiently as you can, and that's what I tried to do . . . He might need IM pain relief tomorrow because he is having a big dressing off his leg and his hand. It should get significantly less and less painful. The first dressing is always the worst after a graft, mainly because it is so hideously stuck . . . If you take the donor area [dressing] right down, it's fiendish.*

On the other hand, there were many reasons given as to why patients should not experience pain, despite their injuries and the potentially wounding procedures performed on them. Deep (third-degree) burns were not expected to be painful, either at rest or during dressing changes, even though patients' experiences did not support this perception. Furthermore, opioids such as morphine were expected to not just reduce but eliminate both procedural and residual pain. Again, this was not borne out in patients' experiences. As their burn injuries began to heal, patients were expected to experience less (and tolerate more) pain, not only at rest but also during dressing changes and, as one nurse expressed it, they should be able to 'cope with just about anything done to them'.

The normative approach the nurses usually adopted towards pain led to constant comparisons being made between different patients, the relative severity of their injuries, and the acceptability of behaviours manifested as the result of inflicted pain. The nurses also weighed specific instances of pain against factors that would either justify the apparent severity and impact of the pain, or provide reasons why the particular pain should not be regarded with concern. Thus a distinction was frequently made between 'real' pain and other uncomfortable sensations that were not defined as pain:

> *I feel the only real pain that she had was when I took the stitches out; she had very real pain then. I also felt there was a little bit of pain following on the inside of her calf around the edges of the graft, because it is quite superficial, and quite often taking that paranet [paraffin impregnated dressing] off it does sting, so there would have been pain then. But it would not have been great, it just would have been an instant thing . . . She did have a little cry . . . I think it was just a sort of built-up emotion. But other than that, I don't think there was any real pain.* (Rose, EN)

Specific patient behaviours were also taken as indications that pain was either absent or minimal. When they refrained from vocal expressions, such as groaning, crying or screaming, or did not complain about pain, nurses took this to indicate that patients experienced little or no pain. When, on the other hand, patients did provide vocal or other indications of pain, nurses frequently defined these as signs of anxiety, fear or even hysteria, rather than pain. In situations where children or young adolescents gave vocal and free expression to their pain, some of the nurses commented that it was the nurses rather than the patients who needed 'tranquillisers or loud music' to help them cope with the stress involved. There were even suggestions that if a nurse could cope with a patient's behaviour, then either there was no pain, or the pain was at an acceptable level and did not require relief.

The following comments refer to a young man, admitted with 12 per cent burns, mainly first- and second-degree. The nurse, Lisa, described his first saline bath and debridement on the day of his admission to hospital. His only analgesic medication was an intramuscular injection of pethidine given more than four hours earlier:[1]

> *Well, I wasn't feeling a great deal then, because he is only a superficial burn. If he was not under any sort of pain control I wouldn't have gone ahead with it, because I can't do anything to a patient unless they are sedated or pain-free. Because it's just . . . it's awful watching someone*

> *in pain. So it's better for me to have them out of pain, and it's also better for them because they are more cooperative . . . I decided that a shower was in order, and he wasn't so badly burnt that he couldn't tolerate a shower, and he was capable of walking because it's only from the chest area up. I could see he was a nice, pleasant man as well, he wasn't obnoxious. So, I assessed all that . . . He only had a couple of lesions that needed debriding, so I knew that wouldn't be painful, and I would have stopped if there had been any pain . . . but I felt completely fine. It wasn't traumatic at all in any way.*

The patient's experience, however, was rather different. Unable to see because of facial burns and swelling, the patient insisted that his wife be allowed to stay with him during this initial treatment. He described his pain as 'hurting' and 'burning', rating its intensity at seven on a scale of one to ten, where ten referred to the most intense level of pain.

When, as in the above example, the nurses made decisions without validating their assessment with the patient, then pain could be made invisible. The patient's restraint of his body and voice, and the nurse's focus on her own rather than the patient's emotional response, allowed the nurse to feel satisfied with her performance, while failing to establish what the experience was like for the patient. Lack of sharing and consultation with patients was one important factor that made pain invisible and allowed nurses to retain a distance between their actions and the patients' experiences.

The first step in the alleviation of pain is not to doubt its reality but to acknowledge its presence. To doubt the reality of patients' pain or to dismiss it as something merely unpleasant or uncomfortable 'amplifies the suffering of those already in pain' (Scarry 1985, p. 7). It also creates distance between the patient and the nurse, making the understanding of the patient's experience of pain more difficult and the alleviation of pain less likely. In the midst of the experience of clinically inflicted pain, adult patients usually try to be cooperative and to retain composure, and they do this by restraining their body and voice (Madjar 1991; 1997; 1998). Thus, the already private experience is made even less visible to others. It is when the nurse believes that this controlled outward expression is the whole of the patient's experience that pain becomes invisible and, therefore, easier for the nurse to ignore and overlook.

Inevitable pain

The nature of patients' injuries and the procedures performed on them in the burn care unit meant that not all pain could be treated as invisible. A young man who screamed during his first saline bath, a woman who cried and shook uncontrollably while her hand was being debrided, a man who cried when he remembered a particularly painful episode—all gave forceful evidence of pain that was severe and overwhelming. Nurses needed to learn to cope with such overt expressions of pain to be able to continue working in this setting. Group values and norms impressed on new staff members influenced how nurses viewed patients' pain and how they coped with it. The working ethos of the unit was that much of the inflicted pain was inevitable and that, except in extreme cases when general anaesthesia might be given, both nurses and patients had to accept such pain as an expected part of the process of recovery, and as something to be approached with fortitude and the will to endure. In the words of Jan, a senior nurse:

> *I think we all know in nursing . . . any sort of nursing, there are procedures that are carried out on patients, that are unpleasant. We know they are going to cause a certain amount of discomfort before you even start . . . It's something that has to be done. I don't ever feel good about it. I think it's something we all have to prepare ourselves for. In fact, before I do a huge, a large burn dressing . . . I think you have to prepare yourself mentally . . . I don't think apart from giving general anaesthetic every time you did a procedure that you can make it totally not painful. And I think that's something that you have to accept, and the patient has to accept.*
>
> *And that's one of the reasons I am not terribly keen on things like morphine infusions, because what I find with morphine infusions a great deal of the time, the patient stays confused and sometimes agitated and disorientated . . . and they are not really, what I would call, facing up to or coping with what in this area often has to continue for a great deal of time [i.e. painful procedures].*

The reasoning in this situation was that opioid analgesics, particularly when administered at more than infrequent intervals, made patients sleepy and uncooperative, and were therefore unhelpful and should be discontinued as soon as possible. At the same time it was reasoned that since pain would recur with each new grafting operation and subsequent dressings, patients would either become 'addicted' or have to learn to cope with pain without the aid of opioids; as they would eventually have to cope 'on their own', then the sooner they started doing this, the better. This is what the nurses and, through them, the patients were expected to accept, and this acceptance was defined as 'coping with the reality' of burn trauma.

Some of the nurses who had worked in other burn care units expressed preference for more rigorous approaches to pain management, but they accepted that such practices were not used in this unit and they followed the accepted routines. Given the general expectation that patients would accept their pain as inevitable, it was perhaps not surprising that patients who were seen as relying on medication (particularly opioids) to endure the pain were seen as not coping:

> *See, [a young male patient] had a morphine infusion until he came here and in many ways I am not sure whether that's done him a service or not.*
>
> (In what way?)
>
> *Because I feel he doesn't cope with pain at all well at the moment. He certainly is someone I would say isn't coping. His burns . . . on the top half of his back aren't that deep. So they will be very, very sore. The area where to me they look to be the deepest, and we are told that there shouldn't be a great deal of pain, he is actually complaining and saying it's the most painful . . . I am not saying that it isn't, but it's just quite an interesting thing.*
>
> (What are you using as indication that he is not coping well?)
>
> *His requests for pain relief, his obvious distress, obvious physical distress, and just his communication, his whole attitude, he is not eating very well yet, those sorts of things . . . I think he is at the stage now where we have to be firm with him, talk to him, try to talk him through [painful procedures, without use of opioids], make him more comfortable in other ways. Try and alleviate pain by sitting him differently, changing his position, and getting him to eat his lunch, and try and think of something else.*[2] (Jan, RN)

While changes of body position or distraction through brief verbal exchanges with nurses were helpful in dealing with some discomforts and less severe background pain, these techniques on their own were inadequate during many painful episodes. Inflicted pain was thus not only *perceived* as inevitable, but in many instances *became* inevitable.

Nurses' perceptions of inflicted pain as inevitable bestowed a form of reality on it—it happened, and it happened within a certain space and time. However, the reality of such pain did not necessarily involve patients' lived experience. It could be, and often was, defined on the basis of the nurses' experience of dealing with patients' overt expressions of pain. This movement from patients' lived certainty of pain to the less solid ground of interpretation of changing behaviours may explain some of the disparity between patients' and nurses' accounts of inflicted pain.

Patients were very sensitive to the quality of the tactile encounter with nurses during painful procedures and, therefore, to the conditional nature of pain (Madjar 1991; 1998). They accepted some pain as inevitable, but were also acutely aware of the extent to which inflicted pain could be ameliorated or intensified by particular nurses' actions. Nurses, on the other hand, tended to see the inevitability of pain as an absolute, and themselves as lacking the power to alter the experience of pain:

> *You could spend an hour and it's still going to be as painful as what you could do something* [sic] *in five minutes. You always are as gentle as you can be . . . and just get them to bear with you. Really . . . I don't feel even sad. Well you do, but you just know that it's the best thing for them, and you know it will only take a week or . . . sometimes it's just the first dressing, and you know it's going to get better. You can get quite hard to it really. Put on a steel face and just do it . . . I think you just get used to it . . . you get immune to it and you just face up [to it] and away you go!* (Nelly, EN)

When the nurses perceived everything about inflicted pain as inevitable, they also saw themselves as unable to change the situation for the better. Rather than seeing themselves as the ones with the knowledge, resources and power to relieve and manage pain, the nurses often felt helpless and immobilised in the face of the pain they had inflicted. Furthermore, the perception of pain as inevitable absolved the nurses from responsibility for its causation. With few exceptions, they felt unable to prevent pain and therefore tried to interpret it as an experience with which the majority of patients could cope, that is, endure with composure and in a way that did not interfere with the nurses' work. At the same time, they interpreted pain as non-harmful and even as somehow beneficial to the patient.

Non-harmful and beneficial pain

The difficulty for nurses in the burn care unit was that their daily involvement with patients in pain continually challenged their attempts to make pain invisible. The perception of inflicted pain as inevitable did not solve the issue either. As treatment procedures were seldom accomplished without pain, the nurses needed to continually justify its infliction, both to the patients and to themselves. Some, as quoted earlier, tried to rationalise pain infliction as something that had to be done, and about which there were no choices. In doing so they had to block or overcome their embodied knowledge of pain as something hurtful and wounding, and construct it as something necessary, non-harmful and justified.

When describing inflicted pain, therefore, nurses did not speak of it as intrinsically bad or as harmful in its consequences, physiologically or psychologically. Having pain was seen as an expected and inevitable part of recovery. The reality of pain was easier to acknowledge when the pain they inflicted was interpreted by nurses as temporary, intense only for brief periods and not taxing the limits of patients' endurance:

> *A little bit [of debridement] doesn't hurt here and there, and that was only a little bit so I wasn't worried . . . She is a good patient really . . . outwardly she seems to tolerate the dressing and the shower and everything well. She doesn't seem to be in a lot of pain . . . I would say she would have sort of moderate pain, but I don't think it would last too long or be too severe.* (Megan, RN)

While some nurses talked in general terms of the benefits of treatment procedures (which had the unfortunate effect of also causing some pain), others were quite specific in describing pain itself as necessary and beneficial, rather than harmful. Such interpretations made inflicted pain not only easier to justify to patients, but also more tolerable to nurses:

> *I didn't like [inflicting pain] when I first started here . . . but I am much better now. I guess it's by having been here a while and seen so much, and done so many [dressing changes]. You know that most of the time they are going to be OK. You don't like having to do it, but it's just something that in the end you've got to do. In the long run they are going to benefit from it.* (Rose, EN)

> *I don't like to inflict pain on people. And I find it quite hard when someone is obviously in a lot of pain. But I've found working here . . . I know it sounds pretty cruel but . . . I compensate for inflicting pain on someone by sort of rationalising and saying that pain will actually help them get better in the long run.* (Kate, RN)

The interpretation of inflicted pain as temporary, necessary, not harmful and possibly even beneficial to patients' recovery was an important means by which such pain was made more acceptable and tolerable to nurses. In turn, nurses tried to use this same reasoning to lessen patients' anxiety and to gain their cooperation. This process of reconstructing pain allowed nurses to gain a sense of satisfaction in their work. They could inflict pain and yet at the end of the day feel good about their contribution to patients' healing.

NURSES' PERCEPTIONS OF PAIN RELIEF

The work of pain management is complex, with changing needs, difficulties in selecting the most appropriate means of pain relief and shifting goals. In the absence of objective measures for any of these parameters, relief of pain can easily become subject to individual nurses' judgements and preferences, and to knowledge and time constraints. There was no written protocol for pain management in the burn care unit and unwritten rules were not necessarily followed. For example, while the nurses often mentioned that patients should be given morphine intravenously prior to first saline bath and dressing change, this rule was often disregarded in practice and some patients received no more than mild oral analgesics.

Minimising the use of strong analgesic drugs

The established routine in the unit was to offer patients milder oral analgesics on four-hourly 'drug rounds' from 7 a.m. until settling time at around 10 p.m. The drugs of choice were paracetamol, a 'cocktail' of aspirin and paracetamol, Panadeine, or Acupan. Any additional pain relief, particularly in relation to dressing changes, depended on the individual nurse assigned to care for the patient on a given day. While there were differences between nurses, opioids were generally used sparingly, in relatively small and infrequent doses (Madjar 1991, pp. 319–25). Often the determining factor was not the reported intensity of the patient's pain, but the timing of the various activities a nurse had planned for her working day. The aim was to make pain bearable, rather than to reduce it to the minimum level possible. The following extract illustrates Nelly's decision-making in relation to a young woman on the day of her admission to the unit with 15 per cent burns, some eight hours after her accident:

> *[At around five o'clock] she said she was starting to get sore again, and that was about the time when she could have had another injection. About four or five hours had lapsed [since her last dose of pain-relieving medication]. So we gave her two Panadol then, only because we wanted to keep the morphine until her dressing . . . Because I wanted to do her dressing at eight o'clock . . . If we had given her morphine at five, given her another lot of morphine at nine, and then it would have been*

> *too late in the evening . . . It took us an hour or so [to do the dressing] . . . Too late in the evening for the dressing.*

The patient's experience was of severe burning pain, yet the medication provided was more suitable for mild to moderate headache or musculoskeletal aches (Fields 1987, p. 272). The morphine that was given three hours later, prior to the patient's first dressing change, was administered intramuscularly and, at 5 mg, amounted to only half of the prescribed dose. It did little to ease the patient's pain.

At 8 a.m. the following day, a similar decision (even though for somewhat different reasons) was made to use a mild oral analgesic instead of a stronger opioid, after the patient again reported severe pain. The patient's previous dose of analgesic medication, morphine 10 mg, had been given at 4.15 a.m. Olive, an enrolled nurse, described how her more direct and specific knowledge of the patient was overruled by a senior nurse's perceived expertise:

> *She said it was getting quite sore again. I had a look at what she'd had. She had some morphine and I actually asked [the senior RN] what she felt I should give . . . She said, 'Try her on some Panadol,' which did tide her over, but we have just given her a cocktail [of aspirin and paracetamol] . . . I would have actually given her morphine.*
>
> (Why would you have done that?)
>
> *I just felt . . . my assessment of it . . . I felt she warranted it.*

Still rather uneasy about going along with the senior nurse's decision despite her own different judgement, Olive justified her deferential behaviour:

> *She is far more experienced at it than I am, so I took her word; we would try that. But . . . I wouldn't leave her in there if I felt that she really did need an injection. Twenty minutes to half an hour later, if she was still in agony I would have done something more about it.*

At least two important issues related to nurses' use of pain-relieving drugs arose from the study: these are captured in their starkness and simplicity in the exemplar above. The first is the ease with which the nurse was swayed to give the least potent rather than the most potent analgesic drug available to a patient in severe pain barely 24 hours after her accident. The second is the more subtle change in the nurse's perception of when administration of morphine may be justified. Initially, the patient's report of increasing pain and the nurse's own assessment of the patient warranting opioid medication may have been sufficient. But once a mild oral analgesic had been tried it seems that to warrant an injection of morphine the patient's pain has to be persistent, extreme and obvious. It was such incidents that reinforced the need for nurses and patients to accept pain as inevitable and something to be endured, and opioid medication as something to be avoided and used only in dire situations. The not-so-subtle message from the senior nurse was that morphine should not be used as the first choice even in severe pain.

Trying mild oral analgesics in situations of ongoing severe pain, however, not only failed to relieve as much pain as could have been relieved, but it also made it more acceptable to use less potent analgesics during painful procedures. The following example illustrates this point:

> *I've given her tonight a couple of lots of Acupan. I don't know if they had given them to her earlier in the day, I haven't actually checked that up. She said that they were quite good during the day. They sort of held her [pain] off. But she was asking me . . . when she had her Acupan . . . if she would be getting an injection, because she had an injection yesterday before both dressings. So perhaps they won't be sufficient . . . I guess I will give her two Acupan [before the change of dressings] and see how they go. If not, we can settle her [to sleep, later] with an injection.* (Megan, RN)

Such 'trying' to see if a milder drug would work meant that patients often had to endure painful procedures with inadequate analgesia. By the time it became apparent that the medication given was in fact insufficient, it was often too late to remedy the situation. Even when opioids were given, the doses were often too small to relieve patients' pain. The following comments by Kate, a registered nurse, illustrate a situation in which the patient was given only half of the prescribed dose of analgesia. The patient was a young man with 25 per cent burns, and the incident occurred four days after admission to the burn care unit. Kate withheld further medication, despite the patient's quite obvious discomfort and pain. The patient's behaviour was not enough to convince Kate that a larger dose (one he was in fact prescribed) was needed:

> *He really did seem to be in a lot of pain . . . I knew it was going to take a long time to do . . . I wanted to give him some morphine beforehand . . . I thought the morphine might help relax him before I take down the dressing and put him in the bath . . . I assumed that 5 mg of morphine [intramuscularly] would have been enough . . . He*

was really uncomfortable when we had finished the dressing and we had returned him to bed. In fact, he was waiting for the next two hours to be over and done with so he could have another injection which would help relax him.

(Why did you decide that you had to wait this long for the next dose?)

Well, he can have up to 10 mg of morphine. I could have given him another 5 mg after the dressing, but I thought 5 mg wasn't effective enough before the dressing, so 5 mg won't touch him now.

Estimations of drug effectiveness

The nurses in the burn care unit expressed considerable uncertainty as to how effective drugs were in preventing, minimising and relieving pain. The small, infrequent doses of opioids given to patients would suggest that some nurses overestimated the effectiveness and duration of action of these drugs. Invariably there was concern about the patient becoming sleepy and 'doped up' as the result of opioid medication and this was often used to justify the use of small analgesic doses. The following exemplar, taken from fieldnotes, relates to a young patient with 25 per cent burns still awaiting skin grafting. It shows the nurse deciding to give less than a third of the prescribed dose of morphine and, despite indications of pain, retrospectively evaluating her decision as appropriate:

> *1.30 p.m.* Patient given 3 mg morphine IV, RN stating that *5 mg would have been too much.* Followed immediately by chest physiotherapy, patient being turned and his [burned] chest being percussed.
>
> *1.40 p.m.* Moved to treatment room for a saline bath and change of dressings. Patient squeezing his eyes and fists tight as moved from bed to trolley. *Sore!* gasped out between breaths. Lowered into the bath. He held his breath and appeared 'winded' as he was lowered into the water. As the RN started pouring water over his burned back his whole body became rigid and his face contorted . . . Mouth open wide and the whole face contorted in a silent scream. Then cried out *Jesus!* Face went greyish-white in colour . . .
>
> *2.00 p.m.* Given oxygen via a face mask. No explanation. The RN is using forceps as a scraper to scrape dead skin and scabs off the larger burns on the arms.
> Nurse: *How is it going?*
> Patient: OK.
> Patient's forehead covered in perspiration. Another nurse supports his right arm while the RN scrapes, picks off and debrides dead tissue.

> Nurse: *Are you warm enough?*
> Patient nods, but does not respond verbally . . .
>
> *2.22 p.m.* Patient raised out of the bath on the metal trolley. Oxygen mask removed. Dried by the two nurses working swiftly. Helped to sit up and large dressings . . . applied to his back. At this point he said he was feeling *faint* and *woozy*. Nurse then asked him to move to a chair [so that she could finish applying the dressing to his back]. He whispered, *I can't*, and was left on the trolley. Face ashen and covered in perspiration.
> Patient: *I can't take any more.*
> Nurse: *You have to.* [No further conversation]
> Dressings to back, arms and foot completed at 2.50 p.m. and patient returned to bed.

In the interview immediately after, the RN stated that she felt that the procedure had gone well and the patient had coped adequately. She considered that the 3 mg of morphine the patient had been given was sufficient and that he did not need the additional 2 mg she had kept on hand 'just in case it was needed. Too much morphine would have made him too doped up to be able to cooperate.' She estimated his pain to have been:

> *not bad, not horrific or anything like that, I asked him if he was OK. If he had said 'no' I would have given him more [pain medication] but he didn't. I like looking after him. He tries to help himself . . . he is doing well.*

There were nurses who, whether they gave analgesic medication or not, remained sceptical as to whether the drugs made any difference at all. They believed either that inflicted pain was such that no amount of any medication (except general anaesthesia) would control it, or that some patients did not have any real pain and therefore could cope without analgesic drugs. Their perception was that patients either did not need or did not benefit from analgesic drugs, even prior to extensive dressing changes. The following exemplars are drawn from a general discussion about pain relief in the burn care unit with two nurses. Their comments relate to a patient with 35 per cent burns who was given no pain-relieving medication prior to a two-hour bath and change of dressings procedure:[3]

> *Quite frankly, I didn't even think about it. You see so much pain relief being used here and, honestly, it makes no difference. Patients still cry and scream and say it hurts, so what's the point? Morphine would have made her sleepy but not really helped much.* (Megan, RN)

> *When she had the morphine she was just zonked out. I don't think she has pain. The way she has been burnt, it's all deep, it doesn't hurt*

any more. It's uncomfortable and an effort for her, but I don't think that it's painful for her. (Tania, RN)

Perhaps because nurses did not expect analgesic medication to make any significant difference in how patients responded to pain, they often assumed that patients had been given all the medication they were prescribed and could safely have. Another assumption was that the provision of pain relief in the burn care unit was more generous than in other areas of the hospital. It was assumed that patients had been given and had taken medication on the regular 'drug round' and that therefore they could not be given further medication even when they reported severe pain. As one nurse, Violet, expressed it:

I think a lot of people do have pain here; I am talking about general surgery, not burns. I think we do quite well with the burns pain relief.

In the same interview Violet also said:

Sometimes you are just about afraid to ask them because you know they are going to say, 'Oh yes, it's still really painful,' and you know you've given them all you can.

Patients who continued to request pain-relieving medication were perceived as relying on drugs to cope with pain, rather than relying on their own resilience and will to endure. The latter attitude was clearly preferred by the nurses, while reports of pain by patients who were seen as relying on drugs (particularly opioids) were treated with some scepticism, or even disregarded. Such patients were considered to be at serious risk of addiction and were therefore even less likely to be given morphine or other opioid medication. Even patients who clearly needed strong pain relief were seen as dependent on drugs, rather than in genuine need of relief from real and distressing pain.

In the case of one young patient, for example, the continuous infusion of morphine was stopped on his arrival in the burn care unit. Skin grafting surgery to his extensively burnt back was postponed for over a week because of his slow recovery from smoke inhalation injuries. Despite daily baths and dressing changes, ongoing severe pain and his requests for pain relief, he received a total of only 73 mg of morphine in small, divided doses over a period of eight days (Madjar 1991, p. 320). This amounted to less than 12 per cent of the morphine he was prescribed and could have received. His own assessment of milder oral analgesic drugs as insufficient during this time was taken as an indication of his not coping, rather than of inadequate pain relief:

> *I gave him an injection [of morphine] one time because he was in a lot of pain; he was really worked up . . . He said he hadn't slept for a good 36 to 48 hours and I could believe that. He was just getting so worked up and couldn't sleep, and sleeping tablets wouldn't work, and no-one was listening to him. Everyone was just saying 'breathe deeply', and he was getting sick and tired of hearing this. I don't think he was really addicted to [morphine] because he said to me that I was the only one who had given him an injection over the past few days. And it's not as if he had wanted it for the sake of wanting it . . . He knew it would relax him and help him go to sleep, at least remove some of the tension that he was feeling at the time.* (Kate, RN)

Even this nurse, however, diagnosed the problem as one of patient anxiety and basic inability to cope, rather than as a situation of inadequate pain relief. Kate went on to say:

> *He is coping with pain a lot better now. I think initially, when he came in, he didn't cope very well . . . I felt that he was very reliant on having the needle, because he said that Acupan and Panadol and nothing else seemed to work.*

The whole area of pain relief was thus fraught with problems for the nurses and patients. Nurses did not feel that the medications they had at their disposal provided the answer to patients' pain. Overall they considered that drugs, particularly opioids, were dangerous to patients—making them sleepy, unable to cooperate and at risk of addiction—as well as ultimately ineffective in relieving pain. The patient's role in pain relief was ambiguous. When patients did not request analgesic medication or give unequivocal evidence of being in pain, their need for pain relief was met inadequately or overlooked altogether. When, on the other hand, they expressed their needs clearly and specifically, they ran the risk of being thought of as not coping, once again failing to obtain adequate relief from pain. The nurses' perceptions of inflicted pain as inevitable and of pain-relief measures as less than adequate required them to develop ways of dealing with situations of pain infliction in their everyday work.

STRATEGIC RESPONSES TO PAIN INFLICTION

The lived experience of nurses in the burn care unit was one of physical proximity to people in pain, people on whom they were required to perform treatment procedures likely to cause further pain. They did not see themselves as having the power to change this situation, either by eliminating the need for the treatments or by eliminating the associated pain. Yet at the same time, these nurses wanted to get some satisfaction from their work; they wanted to feel that they had done something worthwhile for others. To achieve such a sense of satisfaction nurses had to succeed extremely well in reducing the amount and intensity of the pain they inflicted and in maximising the amount of pain they relieved, or they had to distance themselves from the patient for a time, making the pain invisible.

Involvement in a therapeutic partnership

One approach to being in a situation of pain infliction is to enter into a 'therapeutic partnership' with the patient and to work closely together. In such a case, the nurse begins by explaining to the patient what the procedure will involve, listens to the patient's fears and concerns, discusses how the patient can participate in retaining control in the situation, and usually provides some analgesic medication before commencing the procedure. The nurse then monitors the patient's responses closely so that additional analgesia can be provided during the procedure. While accepting that some pain is unavoidable, the guiding principle of this approach is that every effort should be made to keep pain within the limits the individual patient is willing to tolerate at the time. The nurse–patient partnership depends on the nurse's willingness to become involved in the patient's subjective experience, and on her skills in helping the patient to share the lived experience of being vulnerable and in pain.

In the following exemplar, Penny, a registered nurse, makes clear her concern for the patient's subjective experience and her aim of working with the patient so as to share the control over pain infliction and pain relief. The patient was a young woman, undergoing a saline bath and change of dressings to her hand and leg:

> *Initially . . . I felt that she could cope with what we were actually going to put her through in terms of pain level, because I had spent some time with her prior to actually getting her into the shower, and I'd discussed with her what I was going to do, what we were expecting, and the fact that she was going to be in control of the situation. If she felt that it was going to be too uncomfortable, that she could let us know, and that she could take charge. I think that was quite important to her, to feel that she had control . . . I had actually prepared her to let me know what she needed in terms of her pain relief . . . It was really a case of assessing it as we went through it, step by step. I think she coped very well with the shower itself. The hand was a bit more*

> *stickier than I had anticipated it being, so that was actually a bit more distressing for her than I had hoped it would be . . . When she made the statement that she was starting to be uncomfortable with it . . . she was getting a wee bit agitated . . . at that stage I felt she really did need to have some pain relief. So that's where we were at when she had some [more] pain relief*[4] *. . . I think it was important to maintain that trust with her. I had already made the statement that she had control of the situation, and that she was to let me know when she felt it was more than she could handle. I think I could probably have got away with taking off [the final layer of the dressing], but I think it was important when she had indicated that she couldn't cope anymore with what was happening that I, at that stage, went and did something about it . . . perhaps another day it would not have been relevant but today, given the history [of a very painful procedure performed by another nurse the day before], the time spent and her state of anxiety anyway, and the development of a relationship between the two of us, that she could actually trust that what I said was what I was going to do . . . [After the morphine had been given] I felt that we would just take it slowly . . . she was obviously a lot more comfortable, more relaxed . . . so it was just a case of listening to her and waiting for indications from her as to how effective the pain relief had been. I wasn't prepared to go in willy-nilly and assume that because she'd had that pain relief, I could just rip off the paranet [dressing] and we would be set. Because it doesn't always work that way. You don't get total pain relief simply because it's been given intravenously.*

In the above account, the nurse shows acute awareness of the close intersubjectivity between her own and the patient's experience of inflicted pain and its alleviation. Her clinical judgement and actions also demonstrate sensitivity and expertise. This particular exemplar captures best the idea of the 'therapeutic partnership'. In it the nurse accepts the inevitability of some pain, but she carefully works with the patient to ensure that such pain remains within the limits acceptable to that person. Just as importantly, the nurse recognises the patient's lived situation—her experience from the previous day and the resulting anticipatory anxiety, her need to retain some control in the situation and her need to be respected as a person who matters, who can trust and can be trusted. Rather than seeing the patient's anxiety as a barrier to effective pain management, the nurse recognises the extent to which anxiety contributes to the experience of pain, and the extent to which the growing trust between them can relieve the patient's anxiety. Instead of a subject–object relationship the nurse is able to foster a therapeutic partnership with the patient and, in the process, reduce the painfulness of the patient's experience and increase her own sense of satisfaction and accomplishment.

Detachment and objectification

A very different approach to that of therapeutic partnership was also observed. Basically, it involves the nurses concentrating on the technical tasks at hand rather than on the patient. In such situations pain is also accepted as inevitable, but whereas in a situation of partnership the patient decides what pain is tolerable, here the patient is not consulted. As a consequence, the patient's subjective distress is largely ignored and there is little evidence of empathy or compassion from nurses during the performance of pain-inducing tasks. Any pain that the patient experiences is seen as not only inevitable but also as not needing or not able to be treated. The following exemplar, one of a number, is chilling in its acceptance of the inevitability of pain and the degree of detachment nurses are able to achieve in their work with people in pain:

> *Well, I knew what I was going to do. And really, there wasn't a lot of feeling behind it. It was a task and I just set about doing it. I didn't see it as . . . I know it's pain . . . you get her in the shower and it's painful so you try to take her mind off it. You just chat and get it done as quickly as possible . . . You go on not thinking really. You've got your task and you sort of become like a robot. You go in and chat away and take her mind off it while you are doing whatever you have to do. Get it done . . . With adults we just expect them to put up with it . . . they are not going to give them morphine every four hours, or IV drip [intravenous infusion of morphine] for their dressings. It's just not done here . . . If you've got a soft nurse who thinks it must be sore then they are a . . . soft touch, but we expect the patients to put up with it.* (Nelly, EN)

In adopting the strategies of detachment and objectification, the nurses became self-focused, rather than patient-focused. They talked of 'psyching themselves for what had to be done' or 'talking themselves into getting on with the task'. They tried and often succeeded in distancing themselves from the patient's personal experience and from the painfulness of pain they were helping to generate. Often it seemed easier to regard the patient as an object on whom skilled work was done, than as a person with whom a difficult experience could be shared. In such situations nurses inflicted pain, but could not at the same time acknowledge the patient's distress, nor provide comfort when it was most needed.

By contrast, the strategy of involvement in a therapeutic partnership required the nurse to enter the patient's experience and to help create a situation in which the voice of the person in pain could be heard. The patient could thus influence the nurse's body, by having her attention, by influencing the pace of the procedure, by being consulted. The accomplishment of the technical task could be infused with a pathic understanding and become a shared project between the nurse and the patient, each respecting the other's contribution. Within this strategy, the nurse's satisfaction came not so much from a competently performed technical task (although that was important), but from having helped the patient come through the experience of wounding and pain with a sense of personal intactness and control. In the midst of pain there was caring and renewing of hope, the regaining of a sense of embodied self and of a personal future.

CONCLUSION

Nursing education prepares nurses to care, to provide comfort, to ease pain, to relieve suffering. The image we as nurses have of ourselves and would like others to have of us does not include the inflicting of pain and suffering. And yet the lifeworld of nursing practice, especially in acute care hospitals, includes work which often results in pain infliction. It is the reality which the twenty nurses who participated in this study experienced regularly and which they, like the patients with whom they worked, found difficult to put into words. Inflicting pain is not an aspect of clinical work on which we as nurses choose to dwell. It is a source of personal unease and stress; it challenges our self-perceptions as kind and caring people, and it points to our inability to eliminate pain and suffering.

As nurses we can constitute pain infliction into an integral part of our work in many different ways. We can regard it as a delegated medical task over which we have no control. It can then become something that is not seen in its own right and as deserving particular attention. It becomes an inseparable part of the treatment procedure during which it is generated, and assumes the same necessity, justification, inevitability and ultimate benefits. Subsumed in this way, inflicted pain can easily become invisible, and the need for its relief overlooked or not acted upon. Such a view of inflicted pain makes it easier for us to feel no responsibility for our contribution to its generation in the immediate situation. It also allows us to feel no responsibility for the broader search for more effective means of pain prevention and relief.

As nurses we can also regard inflicted pain as a necessary part of treatment, a visible problem only when patients, especially children, respond to it by not restraining their bodies and their voices. Patients' failure to behave in a cooperative manner shifts the burden of responsibility for the pain and distress from the nurse who contributes to it, to the patient who must endure it. Once again, distance is created between the patient's lived experience and our understanding and involvement in it.

However, as research has shown, it is also possible for nurses to retain sensitivity and openness to the patient's lived experience of pain and to our own part in its generation and relief. In such a situation inflicted pain and its relief are constituted into a shared nurse–patient project of managing pain rather than being managed by it. This therapeutic partnership is a way of sharing the joint work of treating the body–subject and ensuring that, on the one hand, the patients retain a sense of control and intactness in the situation, and, on the other, the nurses gain satisfaction and a sense of achievement in their work. The therapeutic partnership is one way in which pain infliction may be openly recognised as an actual part of nurses' work, and which requires its own particular combination of knowledge, skill, sensitivity, moral concern and attentiveness to human experience.

NOTES

1. A distinctive feature of pethidine (Demerol) is its relatively short duration of 2–3 hours (Fields 1987, p. 254). The nurse's comments need to be considered in the light of the type and timing of the medication provided.
2. This interview was given eight days after the patient's injury. Because of inhalation damage to his lungs and the ensuing risks of general anaesthesia, the patient was still awaiting grafting to extensive burns on his back.
3. Although fully conscious, this patient was considered too ill and distressed at this time to consent to participation in the study. She died three days later.
4. The nurse had stopped the procedure at this point and asked that a medical resident administer some morphine intravenously. Within five minutes patient received 8 mg of morphine and after another five minutes the procedure was resumed.

REFERENCES

Fagerhaugh, S.Y. & Strauss, A. 1977 *Politics of Pain Management: Staff–Patient Interaction* Addison-Wesley, Menlo Park, Ca.

Fields, H.L. 1987 *Pain* McGraw-Hill, New York

Gadow, S. 1984 'Touch and technology: two paradigms of patient care' *Journal of Religion and Health* vol. 23, no. 1, pp. 63–9

Madjar, I. 1991 'Pain as embodied experience: a phenomenological study of clinically inflicted pain in adult patients', unpublished PhD thesis, Massey University, New Zealand

——1997 'The body in health, illness and pain' in *The Body in Nursing* ed. J. Lawler Churchill Livingstone, Melbourne, pp. 53–73

——1998 *Giving Comfort and Inflicting Pain* Qual Institute Press, Edmonton, Canada

Scarry, E. 1985 *The Body in Pain* Oxford University Press, New York

nine

On caring and being cared for

PAYOM EUSWAS & NORMA CHICK

The findings of the study on which this chapter is based were first reported as grounded theory forming part of the doctoral thesis submitted by Payom Euswas. For the purposes of the present exercise the same data have been used to constitute a phenomenological description of caring and being cared for. The authors argue that both grounded theory and phenomenology are predicated on an intention to understand the meaning that experience has for the individual person. Each approach requires open and imaginative 'dwelling' with the data so that the voices of the participants are heard above that of the researcher, and both are dependent on writing and the power of words.

The research presented in this chapter was undertaken in New Zealand by Payom Euswas during a period of study leave from a teaching position at a major university in Thailand. Hers is the main interpretive voice which speaks throughout the chapter. Norma Chick, although closely involved as supervisor and mentor, was always at one remove from the initial project. Currently Dr Euswas is an Associate Professor in the Faculty of Nursing, Mahidol University, Thailand. Emeritus Professor Chick, although retired, continues to write and mentor nurse scholars in New Zealand. The authorial collaboration for this chapter has provided an opportunity for insights drawn from their years of clinical practice and scholarly work to be merged with data from Euswas's research.

THIS CHAPTER IS based on research which aimed to identify and authenticate those aspects of nursing practice which best typify caring (Euswas 1991). We believe that caring is central to effective nursing practice and will remain so in the foreseeable future.

In the world of nursing scholarship the earliest concern with caring as applied to nursing is generally attributed to Florence Nightingale, whose efforts led to a distinction being made between the work of professional nurses and that of doctors. Interest in the concept of caring, as evident in associated research, theorising and critique, peaked in the late 1980s. Although the growth rate for related research has slowed since then, and despite the emergence of new critics such as Heslop and Oates (1995), we believe that caring as a key element of nursing practice warrants continued attention. The phenomenological discussion that forms the substance of this chapter shows clearly that the ability to care and to be cared for are recognised by both nurses and patients as being central to their reality.

The core research to be discussed here was designed and presented as a doctoral thesis and published soon after that (Euswas 1991; 1993; 1994). The actualised caring moment is a grounded (substantive) theory that explains how the actual caring process occurs in nursing. It holds that this caring moment is evident when nurse and patient realise their intersubjective connectedness in transforming healing–growing as human beings in a specific–dynamic changing situation. Conceptualised as a gestalt configuration, that is to say as a complex whole, there are three main components of this moment: preconditions, ongoing interaction and situated context.

Preconditions include the nurse, who is personally and professionally prepared to care, and the patient, a person with compromised health and wellbeing. The nurse's preparedness involves benevolence, commitment and clinical competency. Patients are persons in a vulnerable state, requiring assistance from nurses to meet their unique personal health needs. When it occurs as the actualised caring moment the caring process is manifest in the *ongoing interaction* between nurse and patient. The realisation requires that moment-by-moment other caring elements are brought into play, such as being there and being mindfully present, engendering a relationship of trust, actively meeting needs, empathetic communication, and continuously balancing knowledge, energy and time. The *situated context* takes account of the circumstances in which the nurse–patient interaction is occurring. Thus caring, as well as being an intersubjective experience, is recognised as historical and context dependent.

CARING AND NURSING

In everyday life the term 'caring' is used to describe a wide range of involvements, from romantic love to parental love to friendship, from caring for one's garden to caring about one's work (Benner & Wrubel 1989, p. 1). The ubiquity of the term is both a strength and weakness. While it confirms caring as an integral part of our culture, it also works against the aim of finding meaning that is specific to nursing. Dictionaries are similarly broad in their definitions, although there is an attempt to tease out more subtle shades of difference. Perhaps what all the definitions have in common is demonstrated most clearly by the absence of caring. 'Not to care' conveys a sense of indifference, inattention, disregard.

In philosophy Mayeroff (1971) associates caring with personal growth, recognising that through the caring process the carer participates in the reality of the other. For existential philosophers Buber (1958) and more recently Marcel (1981) care in the sense of 'concern for' and 'being present for' is part of their understanding of human existence. The writings of the phenomenological philosopher Heidegger (1927/1962) make a distinction between inauthentic and authentic caring, and bring the suggestion that the meaning of 'Being-in-the-world' is to be found through the realisation that to be is to care. Other philosophical works about caring include Noddings (1981) and Smerke (1988), the latter being a hermeneutical study in which experts from nine disciplines were interviewed about their discipline's knowledge base on human caring.

In psychology care has been found to be a necessary element of childhood development, issuing out of parental love (Erikson 1968). Being cared for is seen as essential to the emergence of the capacity to be caring (Gaylin 1979). Rogers (1958; 1965) identifies non-possessive care as the key to effective therapeutic relationships, while Jourard (1971, p. 201) concludes that in nurse–patient relationships, a well-nursed patient is one who 'feels his nurses really care for him' and senses that the nurse 'tunes in to him at regular intervals to sample his private, personal and psychological world'.

Within nursing literature over the last decade, interest in caring has become increasingly more explicit by those aiming to extend or refine the knowledge base of nursing practice. There is not space to refer to all those who have contributed, since the list extends at least back to Peplau (1952). However it would be reasonable to assert that, with few exceptions, all the theorists cited in what is probably the most extensive review of nursing scholarship available (Meleis 1996) have contributed in some way. Names which are inextricably linked to the study of caring are Watson (1985; 1990), who was able to explicate ten 'carative' factors; Leininger (1981; 1995), who has been steadily developing her theory of culture care; and Benner and Wrubel (1989), who adopted an explicitly clinical focus to caring. As well as the large body of theoretical literature there has been a substantial number of research studies focusing on care, for instance Brown (1986); Forrest (1989); Henry (1975); Hernandez (1987); Luegenbiehl (1986); Ray (1984); Riemen (1983; 1986a); Sherwood (1988); Swanson-Kauffman (1986); Weiss (1984) and Wolf (1986). Some explore the perspectives of nurses while others centre on patients and their families. With the exception of Weiss the studies were qualitative in design.

Of special interest are the studies by Reimen, Luegenbiehl, Hernandez and Sherwood, all of which are described by their authors as phenomenological. They have in common an emphasis on the meaning of experience; the use of unstructured, open-ended interviewing for data collection; and data analysis that follows the procedure which Colaizzi (1978) describes and which Oiler (1986) spells out in more detail. Also warranting special mention are Benner's major studies on expert practice (Benner 1984; Benner & Wrubel 1989) because of both their scope and their phenomenological foundations. As a research method phenomenology facilitates the study of human experience as it is lived. As a philosophy it serves to deepen reflective thoughtfulness about what is important in the taken-for-granted and seemingly trivial aspects of everyday life (Powers & Knapp 1990, p. 106).

It is significant that at the time of Euswas's original research, the New Zealand Nurses Association (the main professional nursing body in the country) embraced, for purposes of their policy documents, the following statement on nursing: 'Nursing is a specialised expression of caring . . .' (New Zealand Nurses Association 1984, p. 3). As nursing research is still in a relatively early stage of development in New

Zealand the pool of other contemporaneous studies was not great. However studies by Christensen (1988), Bassett-Smith (1988) and Paterson (1989) were highly relevant to caring. It may be, too, that a 'circle of contagiousness' (Meleis 1991) affected the spread of ideas about caring. During the 1980s a number of North American nurse scholars including Watson, Benner and Bevis held seminars and addressed professional meetings in New Zealand.

AN OUTLINE OF THE STUDY

Data from which the theory of the actualised caring was generated came mainly from transcripts of phenomenological interviews with patients and nurses, in care settings for patients diagnosed with cancer (principally hospital wards, but also a hospice and patients' own homes). Also included were the researcher's observational field records and memos, as well as nursing and medical notes. Together these constituted the text that was analysed for recurring themes. The questions that initiated the interviews with patients were 'Can you tell me about yourself? I am particularly interested in how patients experience nursing care. What is it like being in hospital?'. For nurses it was 'Tell me about your day', or 'Can you tell me what has been happening to Mr (Ms) . . . while you have been nursing him (her)?'. In both instances there was some guiding of the conversation at appropriate points to ensure that the meaning of any references to the terms 'care' or 'caring' were expanded.

Data analysis followed the procedures of theoretical sampling and constant comparative analysis. In these, 'several research processes are in operation at once' and 'the investigator examines the data as it arrives and begins to code, categorise, conceptualise, and to write the first thoughts concerning the research report almost from the beginning of the study' (Stern 1987, pp. 81–2). The choice of strategy could well have favoured interpretive phenomenology, which 'guides us back from theoretical abstractions to the reality of lived experience' (Field 1981, p. 291). In fact the initial processing procedure closely resembled the pathway for phenomenological analysis outlined by Riemen (1986b). At the time, Euswas (1991, p. 42) acknowledged that what was taking place was a phenomenological transformation of the human experience, whereby 'the person's inchoate lived experience becomes available to him/her in language' and the researcher goes on to transform 'this understanding into clarifying conceptual categories which he or she believes are the essence of the original experience'

(Reinharz 1983, pp. 78–9). In whatever way it occurs, by being given voice the experience becomes more available and comprehensible to both the experiencing person and the researcher. However, a further step involving interpretation is necessary if description is to engender understanding. Here it is presented as the phenomenon of the lived experience of caring and being cared for.

THE LIVED EXPERIENCE OF CARING AND BEING CARED FOR

At the beginning of the chapter we summarised the researcher's theory of the actualised caring moment. This is the researcher's phrase, the words do not appear in the transcripts. It is a transformation, a crystallisation of the many themes and subthemes that run through the participants' descriptions of their experience of caring and being cared for, within a framework of illness. The conceptualisation captured the dynamic wholeness of caring as it had been experienced by the participants. The study provides evidence of the closeness between carer and cared for. It also reveals this closeness to be subject to an ebb and flow in which peaks are identifiable. That is what is meant by describing the actuality of caring as a 'succession of moments'—'moment' is used as a symbol, it does not refer to a set period of time.

The 30 patients in the study were adults, mostly over 40 years old, eighteen women and twelve men, of varying occupations. They all faced some stage of a life-threatening illness—confirmed or suspected cancer. Sixteen of the patients were being treated with chemotherapy or radiotherapy, four were still undergoing investigative procedures and four were acknowledged as being terminally ill. The remaining six were experiencing surgical treatment. Thirty-two registered nurses, all women, also participated in the study. They talked about their understanding of caring as expressed in their practice, and their individual inclusion in the study was contingent upon the fact that they were the nurses associated with the selected patients.

The study began with the assumption that caring is an intersubjective phenomenon. As the data gathering progressed it became abundantly clear that both nurses and patients recognised this condition, and understood that 'being cared for' meant more than just receiving attention to obvious needs. In this sense, caring was an ongoing interaction in which nurse and patient came together in a continuously changing pattern. The nurse is physically and emotionally present, working with the patient moment-by-moment, imparting compassionate intention and physical energy towards improving that person's wellbeing.

As the following excerpts from three different patient interviews show, the experience of being *cared for* by nurses (as opposed to nurses simply being in attendance) hinges on the person's sense of the nurse *being there*. What is so convincing in all the accounts that follow is the admixture of abstract words like 'being' and 'trust' with concrete examples of what is in the person's mind when he or she uses these words. The patients said things like: 'They're usually there when I need them'; 'They're always around you . . . spending time explaining things, talking with you. They're not just doing a job, and then going away'; and 'They are there for a purpose and they do it very well'. Others went further, interpreting 'being there' as a response to their own helplessness and their need to trust. For instance: 'You can't help yourself, you've got to trust them. They know your needs, they know your problems'; and 'Your life is in their hands, so you've got to trust them. They're thinking of you all the time.' Elaborating on the same idea another person said, 'If you feel that they've got your best interest at heart, you're going to be quite confident to swallow that pill, or put up with that thing in your arm, or whatever.' Some statements were compelling in their simplicity, for instance: 'She gave me a good bath. I trust her'; and 'I think trust is the basis of caring.'

Nurses, too, spoke about being there. For one person it was synonymous with caring, caring *is* being there. Others referred to making themselves available, the most direct statement being, 'I am there for them . . . giving them my time.' Just as patients sensed, nurses knew that trust was a key element of any caring relationship, something to which priority must be given: 'the foundation of that relationship is trust'; and 'When I care for the person I need to establish a trust relationship.'

Many of the patients' stories about their experiences of caring nursing involved nurses' efforts to meet situational health needs—physical, psychosocial and psychospiritual. The caring nurse was perceived as one who endeavoured to give the patient control and choice, and made a place for their family and friends to be involved in the care. Recurring themes had to do with sharing information, helping, being an advocate, negotiating, and teaching and learning. Patients commented on the feeling of being well-informed: 'They always explain things to you . . . they ask you and they tell you'; 'They explain the side effects of the medications, what is going to happen, how long my treatment could take.' Patients also appreciated nurses who listened to them. By being heard they were able to establish their individuality: 'I tell them about myself . . . like I am a small eater and I prefer to have vegies'; 'I told them . . . I used to have a problem with my vein . . . I need to have bandaging.' In these examples there is a remarkable consistency with what one of the authors (Hayes/Chick) had found some twenty years earlier, and in another country, when asking hospital patients to describe examples of good nursing (Hayes 1976). Similarly at that time the responses included many things that might easily be taken for granted, indicative of nurses' awareness of individuality. For example: 'That man has asked about his glasses half a dozen times tonight and each time the nurse has shown him that they are safely put away in the locker'; and 'At meal times the nurses always check that the patients have serviettes, and that the meal tray is within reach.' (Hayes 1976) Looked at in this light the cliché 'it's the little things that matter' becomes an enduring truth.

Reciprocity and negotiation

It may seem like stating the obvious to note that caring is most likely to be experienced by those who perceive themselves to be in need of help, but inevitably the receptivity of patients influences their interactions with nurses. This claim does not tie caring to unqualified dependency. What it means is that to feel cared for there needs to be a limit to one's sense of self-sufficiency. This recognition was expressed by patients in various ways, the most explicit being, 'I was hurt . . . I was sick . . . I needed help . . . to me caring was giving me that help.' Others filled in the details: 'They gave me a bed-bath . . . brought my meals to me.' Clearly it is not an automatic 'doing for' which is being described, there is accompanying support and encouragement: 'They listen to what you're saying instead of trying to tell you to do things you don't feel that you are ready for.' Nurses made complementary statements: 'The caring one is the one who leaves the patient feeling strengthened, or leaving a patient in control. A big part of caring . . . is giving back autonomy.' However, they also expected patients to exercise control. For example, with reference to someone experiencing the discomfort of having sutures removed: 'It was up to her to tell me to stop when she needed me to stop.'

Sharing information and negotiation, being an advocate, teaching and learning were other aspects of the ongoing nurse–patient interaction through which caring was demonstrated. Sharing information was not just acknowledgement of a patient's right to be informed of such things as the side effects of medications, and the nature and expected duration of treatments they were about to undergo. There was implicit reciprocity. One patient was able to appreciate this aspect as a shift in attitude that has occurred over time: 'They always explain things to you . . . they ask you and they tell you . . . which is different from a long time ago . . . I was in hospital and they didn't tell you . . . they just did what they wanted.' Negotiation is illustrated in the following extract from one of the transcripts:

> *We had one lady last night that I was looking after . . . She's had a mastectomy and she's got a fungated wound . . . it's quite a deep hole . . . she needs to have it dressed twice a day and she wanted us to bandage it and we wanted to put a breast binder on because we thought that would be better. So we put one on and then in the afternoon she was quite upset. She doesn't like the breast binder and didn't want it at all and so we ended up bandaging her, but her wound was very smelly and that was upsetting her, so we got some powder which is very good at taking the odour away and put that on. Put extra pads on and then bandaged it which is what she wanted us to do, she didn't want the breast binder on so that was a more caring situation because we were respecting her wishes and we were caring about how she felt as a person. It would have been easier for us to keep using the breast binder but she didn't want it so I think we've made her happier in that way and it's been a two-way thing. We've changed our minds and she's told us what she wants, so I think we came to a good solution in the end.*

Although the association with caring was not always made explicit, teaching and learning situations featured in a number of the descriptions of nurse–patient interaction, and provided further examples of relationships that went beyond just conscientious performance of duty. To manage their own care some patients had to master quite complex procedures, such as looking after a colostomy (artificial opening from the bowel), or a Hickman catheter (inserted into a major vein and left in place over the period the person is undergoing chemotherapy). With regard to the latter procedure one woman reflected:

> *I had a good teacher . . . She was one of those teachers that make you feel you had the ability to do it. Some people have that, they can teach you, they don't make you feel that you are stupid and can't do it, they make you feel that you can do it. I think self-sufficiency with patients is important.*

Not surprisingly communication was another major theme. We have adopted the term 'empathetic communication' as a way of distinguishing what is being highlighted here from the ordinary conversation which is an integral part of any interaction, and more particularly those such as informing and teaching. Empathetic communication is not only voice contact—in fact this may be only a very small part of it, or absent altogether. As well as verbal constituents which include listening, are physical touch, emotional touch (through eye contact and facial expression), and other expressions of body language. Each has its own eloquence (we are all familiar with how much can be told or asked with the eyes alone), and in communication that expresses caring all need to be congruent. As well as this necessary congruency within the person, empathetic communication assumes that each person is 'tuned' to the other. A patient's awareness of the nurse's capacity to be able to get 'inside the skin' of another comes through clearly in the following patient's description of nurses working with her: 'Both of them helped me very slowly down onto the stool just as if they could feel what I was feeling, even though that's impossible.' Thus there is work to be done by the participants before such communication is possible, as well as investment of effort to sustain the optimal level of communication. In nurse–patient communication the onus is on the nurse to initiate and monitor these processes.

Euswas later translated some of the patients' descriptions of their interactions with nurses into a series of poems. 'Having a shower' captures a sense of how nurses' simple actions can be significant and empowering for patients:

A big operation, I had
They helped me slowly down to the stool
And gently let me down

They could feel what I felt
'You are doing well' they reassured
I felt good and tried harder

When I went into the shower
I told them I could do by myself
They listened to me and believed me

They let me do it
They're always there
'Are you all right? Are you all right?', kept checking

I felt really confident in myself
I felt I'd achieved a really big milestone
'I can do it'.

Mindful presence

The familiar metaphor of putting oneself in another's shoes was used by several nurses to describe readying themselves to be engaged in the dialogue that is part of empathetic communication. This involves active listening, in which the nurse is sensitised and ready to pick up and interpret the cues provided by the patient. Facing the person so as to facilitate, but not force, eye contact is important, as are modulation of the voice and careful choice of words. Most of these things appear in the transcripts, particularly those from the nurses. For example: 'I sat close to her, I looked at her eyes to show that I understood how she felt. In caring you need to be genuine.' Another said, 'I think touch is one of the biggest things that we use', a sentiment which in a different excerpt is translated into action:

> *I had one lady who was very deaf and of course that makes it very hard to show that you care. But then just putting your arm around her she really sensed that and she hugged me back. She really wanted that contact.*

One woman, thinking back to the comfort nurses had provided when she was experiencing the shock of being told her cancer diagnosis concluded that 'sometimes all you need is a touch. If you're feeling sad or upset all you need is someone to put their hand on your shoulder, or just put their hand on your hand and show that they care.'

Running through the transcripts, showing the many facets of care, is a theme which nurses refer to as awareness, and which we have extended to 'being mindfully present', the essence of which is captured by the nurse who said:

> *I go into the room and ask myself, 'What is happening now and how can I help her? What she needs from me now is this, not that.' You draw your knowledge and experience into the situation at that time.*

Others said things like 'just being aware and wanting to help them' and 'you have to be aware of the moment of being with them'. Even more specific was the nurse who described her thoughts: 'I always put myself in their situation. If I was lying there having that I'd be just as scared. That's how I deal with a lot of my caring.'

Being mindfully present has an even deeper meaning than the quality of being there (for patients). For one of the authors, coming from a Buddhist background, it resonates with the idea of 'right mindfulness' and is expressed by the Thai word *sammasati*, *sati* meaning 'to bear in mind' (Phra-Thepvatee 1988, p. 2). Placed in a nursing context the words imply nurses reflecting on the qualities of caring embedded in themselves, and then translating these into action by being not only physically present, but also fully aware of themselves being involved with the patient they are dealing with at that moment. Connotations of attentiveness and concern come through in this excerpt from a nurse talking about being with patients:

> *I try to concentrate all my attention to them when I am talking . . . They know I am concentrating on them and that I'm not thinking of a hundred other things at the same time.*

Another nurse refers to having 'these sort of antennae, like an insect, that are picking up signals all the time about people'. As well as this direct observation, nurses draw on the verbal and written reports prepared by others in order to augment their pool of information about individual patients, and so be more prepared to take anticipatory actions. That the mindful presence is recognised by patients is apparent when they refer to nurses as 'having the ability to make you feel that you are the only person in their spectrum at that time'.

It is interesting, in view of recent interest in Heidegger's understanding of care, that in this study both patients and nurses chose to explain care in terms of concern. For instance a patient says, 'I think it is the concern that they show for my wellbeing, that's what comes through to me.' A nurse is even more explicit: 'You're concerned about someone and see that they're in pain or that they're upset and you're caring about them and trying to change things, trying to help them.' Walton, in discussing the data from her study of schizophrenic illness, asserts the centrality of 'care' to Heidegger's analysis of 'Being-in-the-world' and notes that for him 'care (*Sorge*) encompasses concern for entities of things in the world, and for other people' (1995, p. 224). She then goes on to refer to 'solicitude', a related term used by Heidegger which refers to a form of care that relates specifically to care for others. These are meanings which permeate the transcript data which we are reporting here.

We turn now to some of the data that highlight the importance of knowledge, skill and professional experience. This comes through in ways that reflect the diversity and complexity of nursing practice, something which demands the continual balancing of energy and time as priorities are set and decisions made. There is recognition, too, that the well of caring is not bottomless, and provision must be made for respite and replenishment.

Knowledge, skill and professional experience

Caring does not occur in a time vacuum. As originally presented by Euswas and outlined at the beginning of this chapter, the explication of actualised caring includes preconditions and a situated context. To reiterate, pre-conditions include a nurse personally and professionally prepared to care, as demonstrated by benevolence, commitment and clinical competency. A strong sense of benevolence and commitment flows from the data already presented.

In real-life discussions of nursing the presence of clinical competence is often assumed rather than asserted. Nurses tend to undervalue their knowledge base, and seem reluctant to talk about it; patients are inclined to take it for granted. For the latter, it is the absence or limits of competence which are more likely to draw comment. A great strength of phenomenological inquiry is that it brings to the fore that which is often taken for granted in our daily lives. Benner (1983) was among the first to illustrate this for nursing practice. This uncovering is not always easy—some of our understandings are so embodied (Merleau-Ponty 1962), so much part of our unexamined self, that they evade scrutiny. Once surfaced, however, this knowledge is available for informed and critical reflection.

It is perhaps surprising therefore that knowledge and clinical competency were such clear themes in our data. To patients nurses appeared quick and efficient at 'administering drugs which takes expertise' and at 'noting that my dressing needed to be changed . . . and it's quite a procedure . . . and then the lines have to be changed every day'. In short: 'Without technical skills they can't really put into effect their practice.' However, as one man revealed, patients were also able to assess differing levels of competence: 'As soon as I got into the ward the nurse checked everything . . . and she knew straight away that I've got infection at the Hickman.' He proceeded to comment on the nurse who had done the dressing previously: 'I guess the district nurse might not have as high experience as the nurse here . . . or she might not see the Hickman very often.' Other descriptions recognise that priority setting is part of nurses' skills: 'You get that sense that once they're qualified longer, they know the important things to do.' That observation is echoed by the nurses who said such things as 'you've really got to decide what's the most important thing', and 'you prioritise in your mind what is most important', both implying that there are time constraints that cannot be ignored.

The nurses were just as forthright as the patients in describing how they understood knowledge, skill and experience to be related to caring practice. For instance, they asserted that caring is 'using a whole variety of knowledge and skills' and having the 'knowledge and skills to help [patients]'. While basic knowledge was not undervalued, relevant experience was emphasised repeatedly: 'You learn the knowledge, but you gain the wisdom . . . experience over the years'; 'As the time goes by you become very much more comfortable with the technical skills.' Further examples were: 'I think a lot of the skills I have been acquiring came by time and experience'; and '*We* also learn from each experience . . . not just the patient gains.'

Although they may not formally think about their knowledge in such terms as empirical, personal, aesthetic and ethical (as introduced by Carper (1978) and extended by White (1995)), nurses realise that their competence depends on an amalgam of many kinds of knowledge and knowing. Effective practice, that is to say caring practice, requires ongoing matching of these personal resources to the time available. The nurses tended to talk about the effects of their knowledge rather than the knowledge itself: 'Knowledge . . . all sorts of effects might not be directly related but it affects the way you think about things at the time.' Two other nurses reflected on their experience when performing nursing procedures:

> *I think about the actual technique, sterile fields and things . . . I knew she was an anxious person, but I didn't know until I actually started doing it that she would be that anxious . . . so even though the knowledge that I had had beforehand . . . you are still renewing at the time that you are doing something.*

> *You have to be really alert to the things that they tell you . . . So if you are going to do the procedure you can adjust it to suit the patient . . . everyone is different, the procedure is the same, but you just alter it slightly so the patient is as comfortable as they can be.*

While knowledge is empowering for nurses, for patients it is the nurses' sharing of this knowledge that brings empowerment: 'They answer any questions we ask and I feel the more knowledge you've got . . . the less frightening.'

The situated context

As discussed earlier, every encounter between patient and nurse has its own situated context which is a fusion of the objective and experienced conditions of the contact. The context incorporates prior experience, but at the same time makes its own demands. Nurses in particular mentioned place and space, as these determined the degree of privacy possible. Several referred to talking quietly and pulling screens as ways of creating an atmosphere conducive to patients talking about their problems. Others commented positively on the nursing philosophies and values of the unit, particularly those associated with primary nursing. Working together as a team and helping each other were also important. As shown in the following excerpt, this had the virtue of freeing a nurse to spend quality time with an individual patient, if she perceived that was necessary:

> *I hand over my work to my colleague by saying, 'I'll be in room such and such . . . Do not disturb me, take a message if the phone rings. I'll be twenty minutes to half an hour.'*

Another factor which influenced what was experienced was whether the interaction was planned, occurring as a reaction to the immediacy of the situation, or entirely spontaneous. If an interaction was planned then the purpose—for instance a dressing that both expected to be painful—tended to direct the interaction.

Nurses were aware that much of their practice fell short of their ideals. They associated caring with time and therefore saw heavy workloads as an obstacle to caring, as something 'difficult in a hospital situation because we haven't got enough time'. Others regarded the oncology wards as a privileged environment, since 'we're quite lucky here, we've got time to spend with patients'. Personal attributes of both patients and nurses were recognised as limiting factors. Not every nurse or patient interviewed described peak episodes of caring, but none denied their possibility or potential benefits. Some nurses spoke of the need to nurture their capacity to care, whether this was achieved through replenishment, such as tapping into spiritual sources, or by conservation, such as learning to 'shut off' when the work day was finished.

The caring moment

The image of caring nursing practice that we have constructed from the words of those who believed that they offered or received it is not precise, but it is powerful. It can be described as essentially a situation-specific dynamic process, which is actualised by nurse and patient as they are engaged in a helping relationship. The caring moments occur within a gestalt configuration that incorporates immediate context and antecedent conditions, the latter defining the nurse's readiness to care, and the patient's need and receptivity for caring. As the caring is translated into the action of helping, nurse and patient experience their intersubjective connectedness. It seems that the more usual pattern for caring is episodic rather than continuous. The actualised caring moment, despite its power, is fragile. The power lies in the potential to bring positive growth for those involved, and for the patient this translates into healing. The fragility comes from our present, limited ability to control preconditions and context. The moment cannot be commanded.

We know that in the course of any illness experience, a caring moment may occur only once and that briefly, despite there being many other similar encounters between the same people. Then again, in the rarer examples it may repeat itself to the point of becoming almost a sustained state. The episodic nature of caring practice is a significant finding, especially in the light of the comment by Barker, in relation to mental health: 'Given the nature of the process it might be difficult for nurses to "care" for long periods of time.' (1989, p. 136). Sadly, at present, we have no guarantee that caring moments will occur at all, an admission that signals the urgency for further research that will clarify both limits and catalysts for caring.

To describe the intersubjective experience—the caring moment—as a gestalt may seem an extreme transformation, even for interpretive phenomenology. However, as was pointed out in the original presentation (Euswas 1991, p. 178) the term, which was borrowed from psychology where it is defined as 'a whole whose characteristics are determined not by the characteristics of its individual elements, but by the internal nature of the whole', is entirely appropriate. We think it conveys the essential quality of caring in a way that prepares the reader to make further transformations, illuminating new experiences as they unfold.

CONCLUSION

The interpretation of caring that emerged from the study offers nurses a philosophical foundation to preserve human caring as a professional value and moral commitment. Darbyshire (1993, p. 57) is in no doubt that such preservation is imperative in what he describes as 'a destitute time' characterised by 'sterile managementspeak'. He insists that 'we must recover our *passion* for and about nursing as a real social force with an ethic of good immovably embedded within it'. On the other hand there are critics such as Heslop and Oates (1995) who argue that the focus on human experience and values leaves us blind to the effects of socially constructed reality (which they imply to be the true reality). Bakan (1995, p. 7) makes a useful distinction between 'literal' and 'real' truth and goes on to suggest insightfully that 'a metaphor or fiction might open a door that cannot be opened by approaches that are too weighed down by duty to literal truth'. In the case of caring the literal truth may be that it defies unambiguous definition—its elements do not reveal themselves under the reductionist microscope, and costing it in healthcare is an accountant's nightmare. However, the caring to which participants gave voice is far from fiction; we believe it to be closer to the 'real' truth. Caring in nursing practice is identifiable, and does make a difference.

REFERENCES

Bakan, D. 1995 'Some reflections about narrative research and hurt and harm' in *Ethics and Process vol. 4* ed. R. Josselson Sage, Thousand Oaks, Ca., pp. 1–8

Barker, P. 1989 'Reflections on the philosophy of caring in mental health' *International Journal of Nursing Studies* vol. 26, no. 2, pp. 131–41

Bassett-Smith, J.L. 1988 'Midwifery practice: authenticating the experience of childbirth' unpublished Master's thesis, Department of Nursing Studies, Massey University, New Zealand

Benner, P. 1983 'Uncovering the knowledge embedded in clinical practice' *Image* vol. 15, pp. 36–44

——1984 *From Novice to Expert: Excellence and Power in Clinical Nursing Practice* Addison-Wesley, Menlo Park, Ca.

Benner, P. & Wrubel, J. 1989 *The Primacy of Caring: Stress and Coping in Health and Illness* Addison-Wesley, Menlo Park, Ca.

Brown, L. 1986 'The experience of care: patient perspectives' *Topics in Clinical Nursing* vol. 8, no. 2, pp. 56–62

Buber, M. 1958 *I and Thou* 2nd edn (trans. R.G. Smith) Charles Scribner & Sons, New York

Carper, B.A. 1978 'Fundamental patterns of knowing' *Advances in Nursing Science* vol. 1, pp. 13–23

Christensen, J. 1988 'The nursed passage: a theoretical framework for the nurse–patient relationship' unpublished PhD thesis, Massey University, New Zealand

Colaizzi, P.F. 1978 'Reflection and research as the phenomenologist views it' in *Existential–Phenomenological Alternatives for Psychology* eds R. Vaile & M. King Oxford University Press, New York, pp. 48–71

Darbyshire, P. 1993 'Preserving nurse caring in a destitute time' *Advances in Nursing Science* vol. 18, pp. 507–8

Erikson, E. 1968 *Identity, Youth and Crisis* W.W. Norton, New York

Euswas, P. 1991 'The actualized caring moment: a grounded theory of caring in nursing practice' unpublished PhD thesis, Massey University, New Zealand

——1993 'The actualized caring moment: a grounded theory of caring in nursing practice' in *A Global Agenda for Caring* ed. D.A. Gaut National League for Nursing Press, New York, pp. 309–26

——1994 'The actualized caring–healing moment' in *Sharing Our Worlds* conference proceedings of the Eighth International Conference on Cancer Nursing, Vancouver, pp. 72–6

Field, P.A. 1981 'A phenomenological look at giving an injection' *Journal of Advanced Nursing* vol. 6, pp. 291–6

Forrest, D. 1989 'The experience of caring' *Journal of Advanced Nursing* vol. 14, pp. 815–23

Gaylin, W. 1979 *Caring* Knopf, New York

Hayes, N.P. 1976 'Interpersonal needs, nursing and performance in nursing' unpublished PhD thesis, Australian National University, Canberra

Heidegger, M. 1927/1962 *Being and Time* (trans. J. Macquarrie & E. Robinson) SCM, New York

Henry, O.M. 1975 'Nurse behaviours perceived by patients as indicators of caring' unpublished Doctoral dissertation, Catholic University, Washington, DC

Hernandez, C.M. 1987 'A phenomenological investigation of the concept of the lived experience of caring in professional nurses' unpublished Doctoral dissertation, Marion A. Buckley School of Nursing, Adelphi University, New York

Heslop, L. & Oates, J. 1995 'The discursive formation of caring' in *Scholarship in the Discipline of Nursing* eds G. Gray & R. Pratt Churchill Livingstone, Melbourne, pp. 255–76

Jourard, S. 1971 *The Transparent Self* Van Nostrand, New York

Leininger, M.M. 1981 'The phenomenon of caring: importance, research questions and theoretical considerations' *Caring: An Essential Human Need* ed. M.M. Leininger Charles B. Slack, Thorofare, N.J., pp. 3–15

——1995 *Transcultural Nursing: Concepts, Theories, Research and Practices* 2nd edn McGraw-Hill, Columbus, Oh.

Luegenbiehl, D.L. 1986 'The essence of nurse caring during labour and delivery' unpublished Doctoral dissertation, College of Nursing, Texas Women's University, Tx.

Marcel, G. 1981 *The Philosophy of Existence* ed. & trans. R. Grabon University of Philadelphia Press, Philadelphia, Pa.

Mayeroff, M. 1971 *On Caring* Harper & Row, New York

Meleis, A.I. 1991 *Theoretical Nursing* 2nd edn Lippincott, Pa.

——1996 *Theoretical Nursing* 3rd edn Lippincott, Pa.

Merleau-Ponty, M. 1962 *Phenomenology of Perception* trans. C. Smith Routledge & Kegan Paul, New York

New Zealand Nurses Association 1984 *Nursing Education in New Zealand: A Review and Statement of Policy* New Zealand Nurses Association, Wellington

Noddings, N. 1981 'Caring' *Journal of Curriculum Theorizing* vol. 3, pp. 139–48

Oiler, C.J. 1986 'Phenomenology: the method' in *Nursing Research: A Qualitative Perspective* eds P.L. Munhall & C.J. Oiler Appleton-Century-Crofts, Norwalk, Ct., pp. 69–84

Paterson, B. 1989 'Making a difference: the lived world of nursing practice in an acute care setting' unpublished Master's thesis, Massey University, New Zealand

Phra-Thepvatee (Prayudh Payutto) 1988 *An Exposition of Right Mindfulness* Bangkok, Thailand

Peplau, H. 1952 *Interpersonal Relations in Nursing* Putnam & Sons, New York

Powers, A.B. & Knapp, T.R. 1990 *A Dictionary of Nursing Theory and Research* Sage, Newbury Park, Ca.

Ray, M.A. 1984 'The development of a classification system of institutional caring' in *Caring: The Essence of Nursing and Health* ed. M.M. Leininger Charles B. Slack, Thorofare, N.J., pp. 95–112

Reinharz, S. 1983 'Phenomenology as a dynamic process' *Phenomenology + Pedagogy* vol. 1, pp. 77–9

Riemen, D.J. 1983 'The essential structure of a caring interaction: a phenomenological study' unpublished Doctoral dissertation, Texas Women's University, Tx.

——1986a 'Non-caring and caring in clinical setting: patients' descriptions' *Topics in Clinical Nursing* vol. 8, no. 2, pp. 30–6

——1986b 'The essential structure of a caring interaction: doing phenomenology' in *Nursing Research: A Qualitative Perspective* eds P.L. Munhall & C.J. Oiler Appleton-Century-Crofts, Norwalk, Ct., pp. 85–108

Rogers, C. 1958 'Characteristics of a helping relationship' *Journal of Personnel Guidance* vol. 37, pp. 6–16

——1965 'The therapeutic relationship: recent theory and research' *Australian Journal of Psychology* vol. 2, pp. 96–9

Sherwood, G.D. 1988 'Nurses' caring as perceived by post-operative patients: a phenomenological study' unpublished Doctoral dissertation, University of Texas, Austin, Tx.

Smerke, J.M. 1988 'The discovery and creation of the meaning of human caring through the development of a guide to the caring literature' unpublished Doctoral dissertation, University of Colorado, Co.

Stern, P.N. 1987 'Grounded theory methodology: its uses and process' in *Nursing Science Methods* ed. S.R. Gortner UCSF School of Nursing, San Francisco, pp. 79–87

Swanson-Kauffman, K.M. 1986 'Caring in the instances of unexpected early pregnancy loss' *Topics in Clinical Nursing* vol. 8, no. 2, pp. 37–46

Walton, J.A. 1995 'Schizophrenia: a way-of-being-in-the-world' unpublished PhD thesis, Massey University, New Zealand

Watson, J. 1985 *Nursing: the Philosophy and Science of Caring* Little Brown, Boston

——1990 'Transpersonal caring: a transcendent view of person, health and healing' in *Nursing Theories in Practice* ed. M.E. Parker National League for Nursing Press, New York

Weiss, C.J. 1984 'Gender related perceptions of caring in the nurse–patient relationship' in *Care: The Essence of Nursing and Health* ed. M.M. Leininger Charles B. Slack, Thorofare, N.J., pp. 161–83

White, J. 1995 'Patterns of knowing: review, critique and update' *Advances in Nursing Science* vol. 17, no. 4, pp. 73–86

Wolf, Z. 1986 'The caring concept and nurse identified caring behaviour' *Topics in Clinical Nursing* vol. 8, no. 2, pp. 84–93

Epilogue

IRENA MADJAR & JO ANN WALTON

THIS BOOK IS addressed to nurses—clinicians, teachers, academics, researchers, managers, scholars—whatever the context in which nurses work and exercise their influence. In it we have tried to communicate what one approach to nursing inquiry, that of phenomenology, has to offer nursing and what thinking phenomenologically—through reflection, research, writing and reading—can do for nursing.

Our intention was not to present either a textbook on phenomenology (a text 'about' philosophy and research) or a textbook on phenomenological research (a 'how to' text). Instead, we have tried to show nurses the value of phenomenological research and writing, which captures the ordinary and the extraordinary experiences of people who live through illness, trauma, suffering and the ongoing challenges that life presents. Nurses are involved in such experiences—as observers and silent witnesses; as providers of treatments and care; as mediators and advocates; as inflictors of pain; and, sometimes, as people who touch the very heart of a patient's experience, and by their understanding and thoughtfulness make a difference. In this context phenomenological description, on the surface simple but often difficult to achieve, is an important means of communicating nursing understandings of human situations. To be able to develop such description (as the authors have done in their chapters in this book), we need to attend to human experience as it is for those who live it and we need to transform it into language that will help the reader grasp not only the events of the experience but also its meaning.

Max van Manen (1990, p. 27) attributes to Dutch philosopher

Buytendijk the idea of the 'phenomenological nod'. In the sense that we, as readers, recognise the truth or the facticity of the described experience—as something that makes sense and to which we can attest because 'we have had or could have had' such an experience—we 'nod' in recognition or in agreement. In other words:

> a good phenomenological description is collected by lived experience and recollects lived experience—is validated by lived experience and it validates lived experience. (van Manen 1990, p. 27)

In the process of inquiry in which the person living the experience is always centre stage, the roles played by the researcher (the writer) and the reader (the wider audience) are critical. The reader in particular is a key link in the process of transforming private experience into consensually validated knowledge (Reinharz 1983), making it personally meaningful and alive.

Phenomenology offers a means of attending to human experiences that lie at the heart of nursing, and the possibility of understanding such experiences in a way that can change how we nurse. To change things, however, we need to understand our own and our patients' Being-in-the-world in a way that is both deep, and true to individual experience.

As nurses we need to recognise the importance of 'pathic' knowledge and 'pathic' relation, which Max van Manen describes in Chapter 2 and which nurses know lie at the heart of what is best about nursing. As nurses we also need to recognise the distress of people such as those with chronic leg ulcers whose out-of-control bodies smell, ooze and fail to heal (as described in Chapter 3 by Marian Bland). And we need to understand the distress of people confronted with invasive technology, closeness of death and a struggle for survival in the midst of critical illness and intensive care (as presented by Vicki Parker in Chapter 4). We need to be reminded of the existential anguish and loneliness of a person with chronic pain, whose continuing quest for understanding is labelled as yet another problem rather than as a way towards healing (described by Ann O'Loughlin in Chapter 7). And we must be sensitive to a different kind of anguish—the need to hold on constantly to a sense of self threatened by the diagnosis and treatment of schizophrenia (discussed by Jo Ann Walton in Chapter 6).

There is a special 'feel' to how Kyung-Rim Shin talks about the experience of Korean women confronted with breast cancer and mastectomy in Chapter 5. There are also universal elements that are recognisable immediately by women from other cultures who experience similar conflicting pulls of personal aspirations and family commitments, and whose personal needs, even in the midst of a serious illness, are often subjugated to the needs of their children and families. Chapters 8 and 9 offer particular insights into the work of nursing—of being with patients in a way that at times contributes to their pain and, at other times, leads to understanding, trust and a special moment of pathic relation. In their description of the actualised caring moment, Payom Euswas and Norma Chick have captured something very important which individual nurses know when they have experienced it but for which we have only a limited language. These writers describe a special kind of presence and attunement to patients and their needs at particular times, which means that even if an intervention is ordinary, its impact may be quite extraordinary.

Each of the writers has contributed a particular reflection on some aspect of human experience of illness. Each has its own particular context and a particular message that readers (if they give themselves time to reflect) will apprehend in individual ways. Together these reflections are not exhaustive, but they are true to the human struggle for health, for recovery, for understanding and for meaning. We hope that in reading this book, readers will be challenged not only to read the text but to be read by it—to reflect on their experience and their practice in the light of the ideas presented. We hope that the reading will help you to see the experience of illness and of nursing in a fresh way.

REFERENCES

Reinharz, S. 1983 'Phenomenology as a dynamic process' *Phenomenology + Pedagogy* vol. 1, no. 1, pp. 77–9

van Manen, M. 1990 *Researching Lived Experience: Human Science for an Action Sensitive Pedagogy* Althouse Press, London, Ontario

Index